THE BOOK OF

CHILDREN'S FOODS

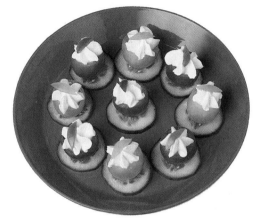

T H E   B O O K   O F

CHILDREN'S FOODS

LORNA RHODES

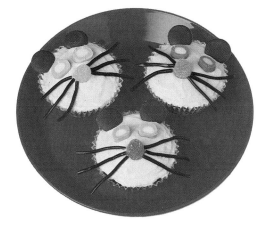

Photographed by
SUE JORGENSEN

HPBooks
a division of
PRICE STERN SLOAN
Los Angeles

ANOTHER BEST SELLING VOLUME FROM HPBOOKS

HPBooks
A division of Price Stern Sloan, Inc.
11150 Olympic Boulevard
Suite 650
Los Angeles, California 90064
9 8 7 6 5 4 3 2 1

By arrangement with Salamander Books Ltd.

Home Economist: Lorna Rhodes
Printed in Belgium by Proost International Book Production

CONTENTS

INTRODUCTION

Cooking for children can be fun. They love brightly-colored food and are often happy with the most simple creations. In our ever-changing world, however, children are exposed to a wider variety of food than ever before—indeed, many are fortunate enough to have traveled with their parents and sampled foreign dishes. Gone are the days when schoolchildren were given nursery food as a matter of course; now they often also like many of the sophisticated dishes their parents enjoy.

As parents we are responsible for giving children the best start possible in life, and an important contribution to this aim is making available wholesome, fresh foods. A balanced diet is important for everyone, but starting children off with good eating patterns and encouraging them to eat plenty of fruit and vegetables, and less fatty foods, is the best investment we can make for their future health.

This book has a wide selection of recipes for children of all ages, with enticing dishes for preschoolers, plus grown-up ideas for older children. Older children, who enjoy cooking, can make many of the recipes with parental approval. The recipes are easy to follow, especially with the help of the step-by-step photographs. Older children will also love helping prepare the fun ideas for younger brothers and sisters, especially when it's for a birthday party or a special treat. Most of the recipes have been chosen with everyday eating in mind, but there are also delicious treats and desserts for those special celebrations.

It often seems an easy option to choose commercially prepared food, such as fish sticks and hamburgers, for the family, but what could be nicer and more wholesome than homemade baked fish or a freshly made pasta dish? The recipes included help offer lots of interesting ideas for healthy meals, using the foods children enjoy.

With over 100 delicious recipes, all photographed in full color and with step-by-step directions, this book will appeal to people of all ages who love cooking and eating delicious food.

FOOD FOR CHILDREN

Food for children should be fun, with family meals a pleasant and relaxed occasion. Yet it is equally important that children learn to enjoy the taste of fresh and wholesome foods at an early age. This can easily be achieved by presenting food in novel and unusual ways. Cutting food into shapes, such as stars and animals, numbers and letters, will certainly interest young children, and foods which can be eaten with the fingers, such as pizzas, pita bread and corn-on-the-cob are always popular.

HEALTHY EATING

Healthy eating is all about providing the right kind of food in a balanced way, so the wholesome and natural ingredients can be enjoyed while they provide the vital nutrients necessary for children's growth and maintenance. Food should be fun, and for children this can be quite easy to do. Encourage them to eat plenty of fresh fruit and vegetables; children are attracted by the bright colors of the many varieties available. Offer a varied selection, and introduce tropical fruits as a treat to interest them in new tastes and textures. Most fruits and vegetables can be cut into easy-to-eat sizes, which is a good way of serving food to young children. Chunks of apple, carrot and cucumber are great snack foods for children of all ages.

Try to use unrefined ingredients and food rich in starch and fiber, such as potatoes, rice, pasta and grains. Limit the intake of refined food, especially sugar. Growing children need plenty of energy, which can be provided by starchy foods, but do not fall into the trap of offering too much fatty or sugary food. Not only will they miss out on other nutrients, but many children can become obese by snacking on potato chips, French fries, cookies and candies. Overweight children with bad eating habits tend to exercise less, setting a pattern that will lead them to all sorts of health problems later in life.

Children's teeth are at risk from tooth decay, but forbidding candy at a young age will only make it more attractive. Reduce the damage by limiting candy to a certain time, such as at the end of a meal, and offer candy as a treat, rather than part of everyday eating. Do not use candy as a reward to comfort an unhappy child. Young children especially can be very manipulative with tantrums, and it is all too easy to placate a child with candy. Avoid giving children carbonated drinks laden with sugar. Remember to dilute fruit juice with mineral water, as it is quite high in natural sugar. Choose breakfast cereals with little or no added sugar. Baby foods and drinks do not need added sugar.

CHILDREN'S TASTES

Children's tastes often go in phases of likes and dislikes. One day a child may hate cheese, then suddenly the next day, he or she will adore cheese-topped pizzas. They may also have a passion for dishes that are not necessarily the healthiest. Fatty hamburgers and hot dogs, for example, are often favorite foods. So either make your own with very lean meats or buy low-fat varieties, and broil rather than fry. Similarly, broil or bake fish sticks. It is also a good idea to cut down on animal sources of fat such as butter, full-fat cheeses and red meat.

Very young children rely on milk as the main food for most of their calories. Children under two years need whole milk, then they can drink low-fat milk. Homemade milk shakes with no added sugar make nutritious drinks. Small cartons of low-fat yogurt, available at supermarkets, are easy to eat and make excellent snacks or desserts for small children. Be sure you read the label, however, and buy brands that do not have high sugar contents.

Remember that children's appetites vary greatly. They often prefer smaller meals and snacks throughout the day and can be put off by larger meals. In this book, there are plenty of recipe ideas for both main meals, as well as healthy snack foods. The portions are a guideline, as much will depend on the age of the children being fed. Often a 10 year old can eat twice as much as a seven year old, and as a child becomes a teenager, it sometimes seems they are continually hungry.

CHILDREN & THE FAMILY

With today's busy lifestyles, most children's meals will be the family's meals as well. For mothers at home with young children, the recipes in this

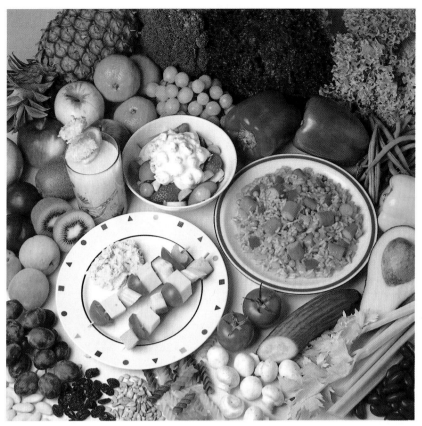

book provide lots of new and attractive ideas. But for working mothers there is rarely enough time to cook children's food separately. It is important that the food chosen for family meals is appealing to everyone, with an emphasis on healthy ingredients. Many of the recipes in the Suppers & Lunches chapter can be enjoyed by both children and adults. In general, children just eat smaller versions of adult meals. If we want our children to grow up with good eating habits, it is important for parents to set an example by eating the right kinds of foods when sharing family meals with their children.

General guidelines apply when shopping for all ages. Read the labels on foods to check that they are low in fat. Keep a supply of quick-cooking, low-fat foods, such as fish fillets and chicken pieces, in the freezer.

Avoid frying—broil, steam or bake with minimal fat or use a microwave oven because of the less fat needed for microwave cooking. Use oil or fat sparingly. Choose an oil high in polyunsaturated fatty acids, such as safflower or soy bean, or a polyunsaturated margarine—one in which the liquid vegetable oil is listed first on the label. When a baby or younger child is sharing the family food, it is best not to add salt, pepper or spices. These can always be added at the table.

Take advantage of labor-saving kitchen equipment such as the food processor and microwave oven. Microwave ovens work quickly, enabling you to produce quick snacks. Microwave ovens cook foods with a minimal amount of water, preventing unnecessary loss of nutrients.

VEGETARIAN IN THE FAMILY

An increasing number of people are eating vegetarian meals, including many children who choose to become vegetarians. A parent whose child chooses to be a vegetarian will need to learn how to combine foods, such as beans and grains, to achieve a first-class protein intake, and protein-rich meat alternatives like tofu made from soybeans. A family diet can be altered to suit a vegetarian child and remain very healthy, with the emphasis on whole foods, grains and seeds. Vegetable burgers and patties and vegetarian sausages, for example, are not just for vegetarians. They can add variety to the diet and can be enjoyed by the whole family. There are several recipes throughout the book which do not use meat, yet they are still attractive, fun and nutritious.

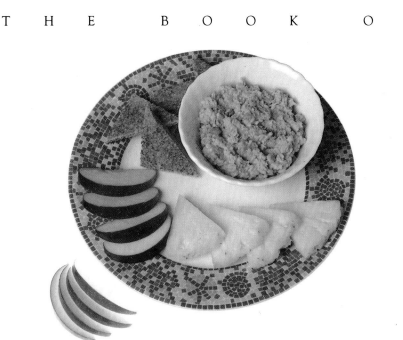

BREAKFAST DIP

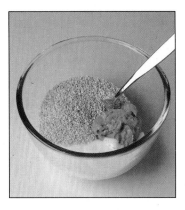

1/2 cup crunchy peanut butter
2 tablespoons sesame seeds
6 tablespoons low-fat plain yogurt
2 thick slices bread
2 apples
1/2 small pineapple

Into a bowl, put peanut butter, sesame seeds and yogurt. Mix together until well blended.

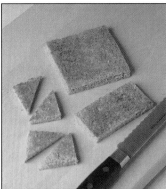

Toast the bread, then cut off crusts and cut each slice into 8 triangles.

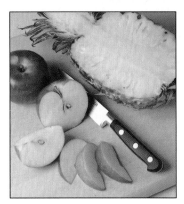

With a sharp knife, quarter apples, remove cores and cut each piece into 3 slices. Cut skin off pineapple and discard. Cut pineapple into small wedges. Serve the dip with toast and fruit.

Makes 4 to 6 servings.

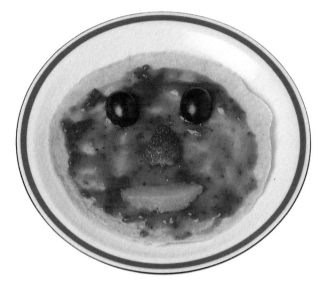

FRUITY CREPE FACES

1/2 cup whole-wheat flour
1/2 cup all-purpose flour
2 eggs, beaten
1-1/4 cups milk
1 orange
4 strawberries
8 grapes
4 tablespoons reduced-sugar jam
2 tablespoons butter

Into a bowl, put flours. Make a well in center, add the eggs and milk and beat to form a smooth batter.

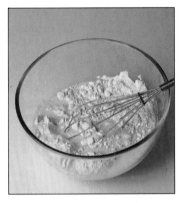

Let batter stand while preparing fruit. Peel and section the orange; halve strawberries and grapes, removing seeds from grapes, if needed. Into a small saucepan, put jam. Warm gently to soften. To make crepes, heat a 5-inch skillet over medium-high heat. Melt a little butter in pan (just enough to coat the surface).

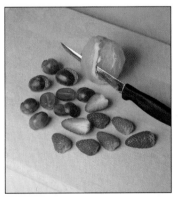

Pour in enough batter to cover bottom of pan (about 1/4 cup). Cook until batter is no longer runny and underside is lightly browned. With a metal spatula, turn over crepe and cook 30 to 45 seconds. Slide crepe onto a plate and keep warm while cooking remaining batter. To serve, spread a spoonful of jam over each crepe, place an orange section for the mouth, a strawberry half for the nose and grape halves for eyes.

Makes 8 crepes.

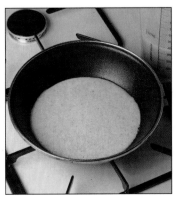

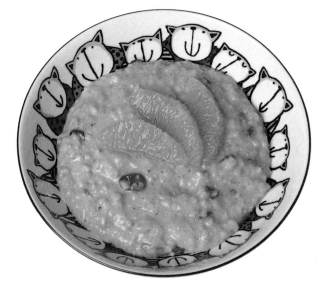

BREAKFAST SURPRISE

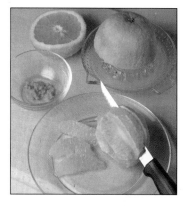

2 large oranges
1-1/3 cups quick-cooking rolled oats
2 cups milk
1/3 cup dark or golden raisins
1 tablespoon honey

Grate zest from 1 orange and squeeze out juice. Remove peel and white pith from remaining orange and cut into sections; set aside.

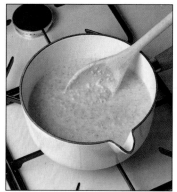

Into a medium-size saucepan, put orange zest and juice, oats and milk. Bring to a boil, stirring constantly. Reduce heat to low and cook 1 minute.

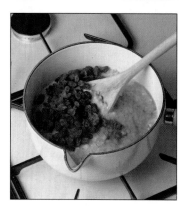

Stir in raisins and honey. Divide among 4 serving bowls and decorate each with orange sections. Serve at once.

Makes 4 servings.

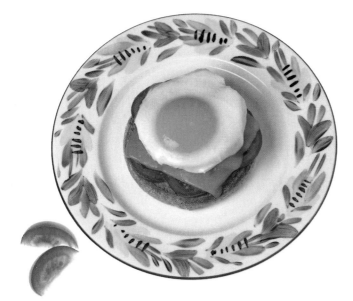

EGG & CHEESE MUFFINS

2 whole-wheat English muffins
Margarine, softened
2 large tomatoes, sliced
4 slices Cheddar or Edam cheese
4 eggs

Preheat broiler. With a sharp knife, cut muffins in half. Lightly toast, then spread with a little margarine.

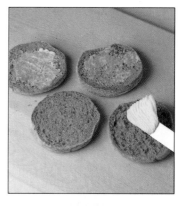

Divide tomato slices among muffin halves and place a cheese slice on top of each. Broil until cheese is just beginning to melt.

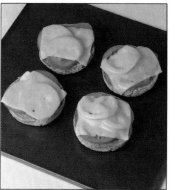

Meanwhile, into a large skillet, pour about 1 inch of water. Bring to a simmer. Break each egg into water and poach over medium heat until the whites are firm and yolks set. Lift out with a slotted spoon and place an egg on each muffin half. Serve at once.

Makes 4 servings.

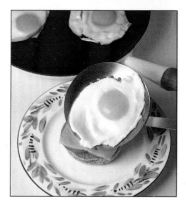

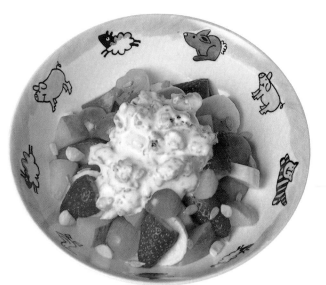

—FRUITY MORNING STARTER—

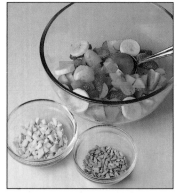

4 ounces strawberries
4 ounces seedless grapes
1 peach or nectarine or 2 plums
1 banana
2 tablespoons almonds, coarsely chopped
1 tablespoon sunflower seed kernels
5 tablespoons plain low-fat yogurt
2 teaspoons honey
3 tablespoons crunchy oat cereal

Rinse, cap and halve strawberries. Halve the grapes. Peel and dice peach. Slice banana. Into a bowl, put prepared fruit and mix together.

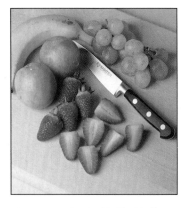

Add almonds and sunflower kernels to fruit. Mix lightly together, then divide among 4 serving dishes.

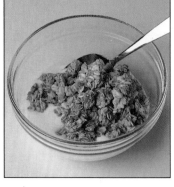

Mix yogurt with honey and stir in the cereal. Spoon over fruit to serve.

Makes 4 servings.

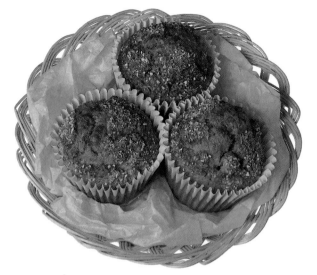

———— BANANA MUFFINS ————

1 cup all-purpose flour
1 cup whole-wheat flour
1 tablespoon baking powder
1/2 cup regular rolled oats
1/3 cup packed light brown sugar
1/2 cup walnuts, finely chopped
2 eggs
1/4 cup honey
2/3 cup milk
3 tablespoons vegetable oil
1/2 teaspoon vanilla extract
2 ripe bananas
TO FINISH:
2 teaspoons regular rolled oats and 2 teaspoons brown
    sugar

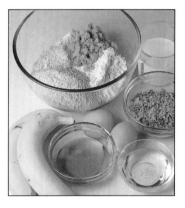

Preheat oven to 400F (205C). Into a bowl, sift flours and baking powder. Add any bran remaining in the sifter. Stir in oats, sugar and nuts. In another bowl, beat together eggs, honey, milk, oil and vanilla extract. Add to dry ingredients and stir just until blended. Mash bananas, then stir into batter.

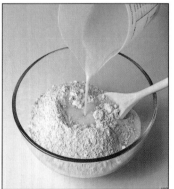

Divide batter among 12 paper cupcake cups in a 12-cup muffin pan. Mix the 2 teaspoons oats and 2 teaspoons brown sugar together and scatter over the top of the muffins. Bake 20 to 25 minutes, until golden. Serve warm.

Makes 12.

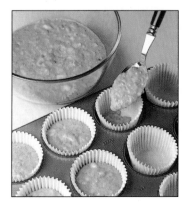

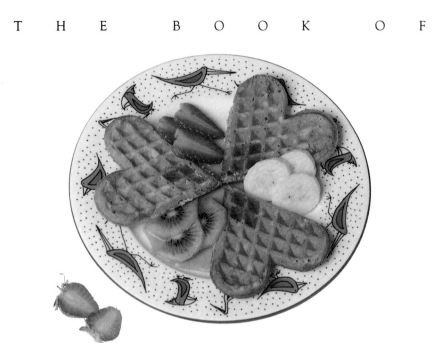

OAT WAFFLES

1 cup all-purpose flour
1 cup whole-wheat flour
2/3 cup regular rolled oats
1/3 cup packed light brown sugar
2 teaspoons baking powder
1/2 teaspoon salt
2 eggs
1-1/2 cups milk
2 tablespoons vegetable oil plus extra for cooking

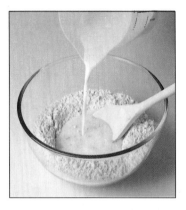

Heat a waffle iron according to the manufacturer's directions. Into a bowl, put flours, oats, sugar, baking powder and salt. In another bowl, beat together eggs, milk and oil. Add to dry ingredients.

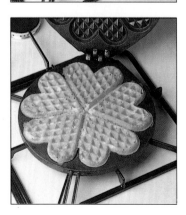

Using a wooden spoon, stir ingredients together just until combined. Brush the grids of the waffle iron with a little oil. Ladle enough batter onto the preheated surface to cover about two-thirds.

Close lid and cook waffles until crisp and golden and steam no longer comes from the waffle iron. Serve the waffles at once, topped with yogurt or maple syrup and fresh fruit or a fruit puree.

Makes about 5 waffles or 20 squares.

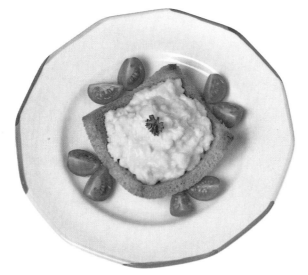

SCRAMBLED EGG CUPS

1/4 cup butter
4 large slices bread, crusts removed
4 eggs
2 tablespoons milk
Salt and pepper
1/4 cup shredded Cheddar cheese (1 ounce)
Tomato wedges and parsley sprigs, to garnish

Preheat oven to 400F (205C). In a small saucepan, melt half the butter. Brush both sides of each bread slice with the melted butter.

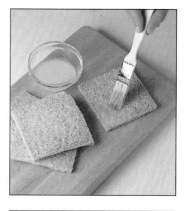

Line 4 (3-inch) quiche pans with the bread slices, pressing them down well in the center but leaving the corners pointing up. Bake 15 to 20 minutes, until crisp and golden.

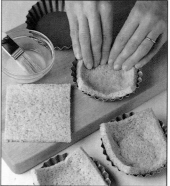

About 5 minutes before the bread cups are ready, in a medium-size bowl, beat eggs and milk together. Stir in salt, pepper and cheese. In a small saucepan, melt remaining butter and pour in the egg mixture. Cook over low heat, stirring constantly, until eggs are set but still creamy. Remove from heat, spoon into the bread cups and serve immediately. Garnish with tomato wedges and parsley sprigs.

Makes 4 servings.

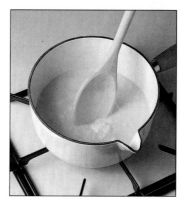

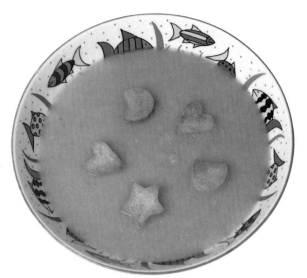

SUNSHINE SOUP

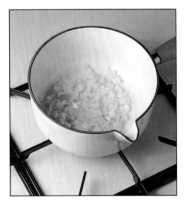

1 tablespoon butter or margarine
1 small onion, finely chopped
2 cups chopped carrots
2 tablespoons red lentils
2-1/2 cups vegetable stock
Juice of 1 small orange
CROUTONS:
2 slices bread
Vegetable oil for frying

In a medium-size saucepan, melt butter. Add onion and cook until softened, stirring occasionally.

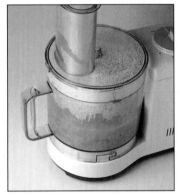

Stir in carrots and lentils, then pour in stock. Bring to a boil, reduce heat and simmer 15 to 20 minutes, until carrots are tender. Process in a blender or food processor fitted with the metal blade until very smooth.

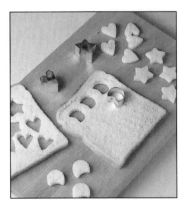

Return mixture to pan and reheat. Stir in orange juice. Keep warm. To make croutons, with very small cookie cutters, cut out shapes from bread. In a skillet, heat a little oil and cook bread shapes until golden. Drain on paper towels and serve as a garnish with the soup.

Makes 4 to 5 servings.

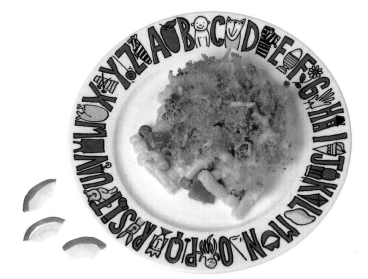

RAINBOW MACARONI & CHEESE

3/4 cup macaroni
6 tablespoons all-purpose flour
1-1/4 cups milk
1 tablespoon butter or margarine
Salt and pepper
1/3 cup frozen green peas
1/3 cup frozen whole-kernel corn
1 tomato, diced
3/4 cup shredded Gouda or Edam cheese (3 ounces)
1/2 cup whole-wheat bread crumbs

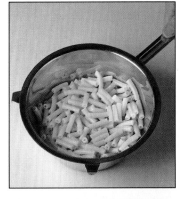

Cook macaroni in boiling salted water according to package directions until just tender to the bite. Drain.

In a medium-size saucepan, combine flour and a little of the milk until smooth. Gradually stir in remaining milk; add butter. Cook over medium heat, stirring constantly, until thickened. Season with a little salt and pepper. Reduce heat to low and add peas, corn, tomato and 1/2 cup of the cheese. Cook, stirring, 2 minutes. Meanwhile, preheat broiler.

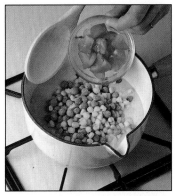

Stir in macaroni and heat through. Spoon mixture into 4 small ovenproof dishes or 1 large one. Mix together bread crumbs and remaining cheese, then sprinkle on top of macaroni mixture. Place under hot broiler 3 to 4 minutes, until browned. Serve immediately.

Makes 4 servings.

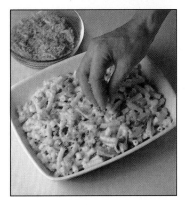

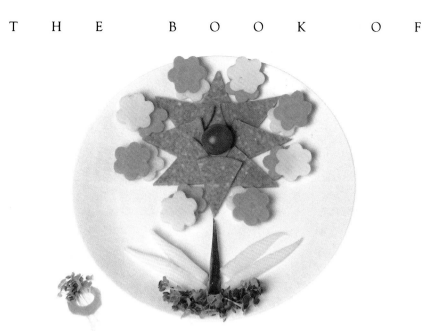

──CHILDREN'S ANTIPASTO──

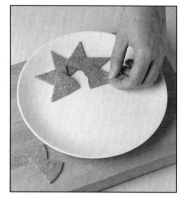

4 slices mild salami or ham
2 cherry tomatoes
4 slices mild cheese
2 large carrots, sliced
2-inch piece cucumber
Radish or mustard sprouts

With a knife, cut each salami slice into quarters. Divide between 2 plates, arranging salami slices in a circle with the points facing out. Place 1 tomato in center of each.

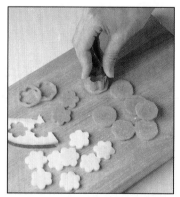

Using a small flower cookie cutter, cut out shapes from cheese. (The trimmings can be used for a sauce.) Cut out flowers from the carrot slices as well. Arrange with cheese around the edge of the plate to look like flower petals.

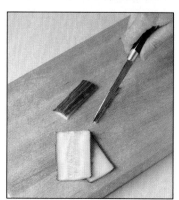

With a knife, cut a long slice of cucumber, then cut 2 thin strips to resemble stems for the flowers. Cut long slices from remaining cucumber and shape them to look like leaves. Place 4 on each flower. Snip sprouts and arrange on plate to look like grass.

Makes 2 servings.

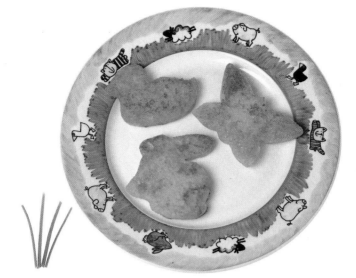

ZOO FRENCH TOAST

6 slices bread
1 large egg
3 tablespoons milk
3 tablespoons butter

With cookie cutters, cut bread into animal shapes.

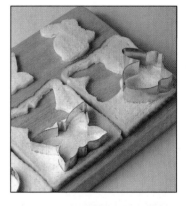

In a shallow dish, beat egg and milk together.

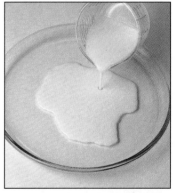

In a large skillet, melt butter. Dip bread shapes in egg mixture, coating each side. Place egg-coated shapes in skillet and cook on each side until golden. Serve at once.

Makes about 12 pieces.

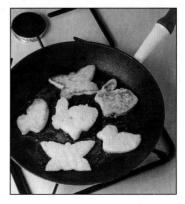

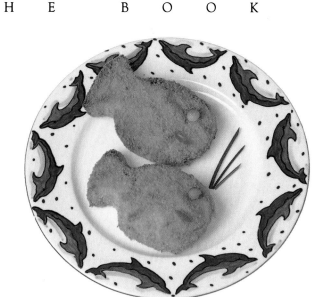

FUN FISH CAKES

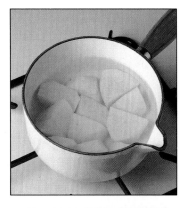

1/2 pound potatoes, peeled
Salt
2 tablespoons butter or margarine
1 egg yolk
1 tablespoon snipped fresh chives
1 (7-oz.) can tuna in water, drained
1 egg, beaten
3/4 cup dry bread crumbs
Vegetable oil for cooking
4 green peas
1 small tomato
Fresh chives, to garnish

Preheat the oven to 400F (205C). Grease a baking sheet. Cut the potatoes into pieces.

In a pan of lightly salted boiling water, boil potatoes just until tender. Drain potatoes. Return to pan and dry over low heat a few moments. Add butter and egg yolk, then mash together. Stir in chives and tuna. Divide mixture into 6 equal portions. With floured hands, shape portions into flat pear shapes. Shape the thinner end of the fish cakes to form a V-shape, like the tail of a fish.

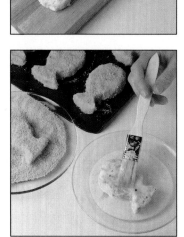

Into a shallow dish, put beaten egg. Gently add fish cakes to egg and brush tops with egg. Coat in bread crumbs, then place on baking sheet. Brush with a little oil. Bake 20 to 25 minutes, until crisp and golden. To serve, place a pea on each fish for an eye and add a small sliver of tomato for the mouth. Garnish with chives and serve hot.

Makes 6 servings.

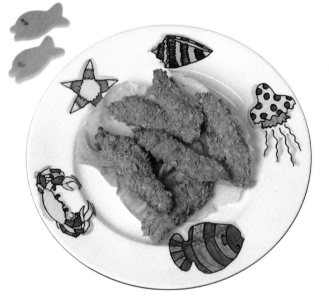

FISH FLIPS

Vegetable oil
2 flounder fillets, each weighing about 10 ounces,
    skinned
2 tablespoons all-purpose flour
Salt and pepper
1 egg, beaten
3 cups cornflakes, crushed
Lettuce leaves, to serve

Preheat oven to 375F (190C). Grease 2 baking sheets with oil. Cut flounder fillets into 24 (1-inch-wide) strips.

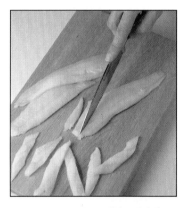

Season flour with salt and pepper. Into a shallow dish, put beaten egg. Dust fish strips in flour, then dip into beaten egg.

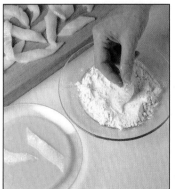

Coat fish strips in crushed cornflakes, then place on baking sheets. Bake 15 minutes, until coating is crisp. To serve, place lettuce leaves on 4 plates. Arrange 6 fish strips on each plate.

Makes 4 servings.

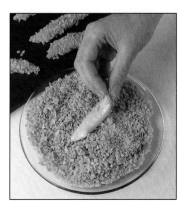

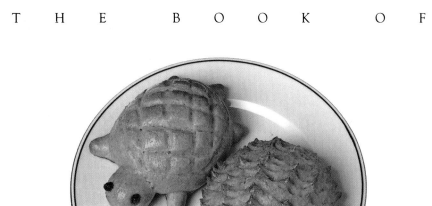

——— ANIMAL BREAD ROLLS ———

2 cups whole-wheat flour
2 cups bread flour
1 (1/4-oz.) package active dry yeast
Pinch of salt
1 tablespoon vegetable oil
2 teaspoons honey
1-1/4 cups warm water (130F, 55C)
Dried currants, to decorate
1 egg, beaten

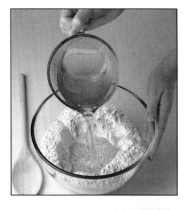

Grease 2 baking sheets. In a large bowl, put flours, yeast and salt. Make a well in the center. Mix oil with honey and water, then pour into well.

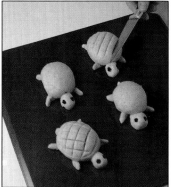

Mix to form a stiff dough. Turn dough out onto a floured surface and knead. Divide into 8 pieces. From each of 4 pieces, take a small piece to form a tail and 4 feet and a slightly larger piece for the head, leaving remaining dough for body. Shape body piece into a ball and flatten slightly. Shape and attach small pieces to look like feet and tail. Attach larger piece for head and place 2 currants in position for eyes. Transfer to a baking sheet. With a sharp knife, mark top of body in crisscross pattern, to look like a tortoise shell.

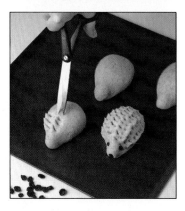

With remaining 4 pieces of dough, shape each into an oval with a pointed end. Transfer to a baking sheet. Using sharp scissors, snip tops to look like spines on porcupines and insert currants for eyes and nose. Cover with plastic wrap and let rise in a warm place 30 minutes, until almost doubled in size. Preheat oven to 450F (230C). Brush rolls with beaten egg. Bake 15 to 20 minutes, until cooked through and golden-brown.

Makes 8.

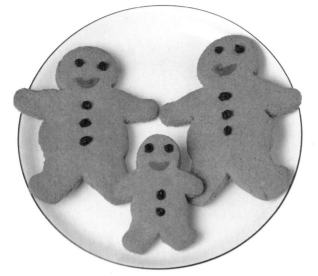

GINGERBREAD FRIENDS

1-3/4 cups whole-wheat flour
1 teaspoon baking soda
1 teaspoon ground cinnamon
1 teaspoon ground ginger
6 tablespoons margarine
3/4 cup packed light brown sugar
2 tablespoons light corn syrup
1 tablespoon orange juice
Dried currants and candied cherries, to decorate

Preheat oven to 325F (165C). Grease 2 baking sheets. Into a medium-size bowl, place flour, then sift in baking soda and spices.

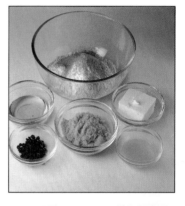

Into a saucepan, put margarine, sugar and corn syrup, then heat, stirring, until melted. Cool mixture, then pour onto the flour. Add orange juice and mix to a firm dough.

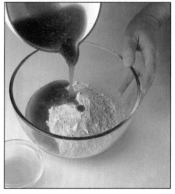

Turn dough out onto a floured surface. Roll out to about 1/4 inch thick. Using people-shaped cookie cutters, cut out gingerbread men and women. Place cookies on baking sheets. Decorate with currants and slivers of candied cherry. Bake 15 minutes, until firm. Cool slightly, then transfer to a wire rack to cool completely. Store in an airtight container.

Makes 8 to 10.

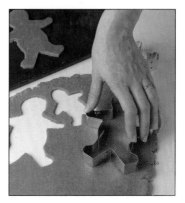

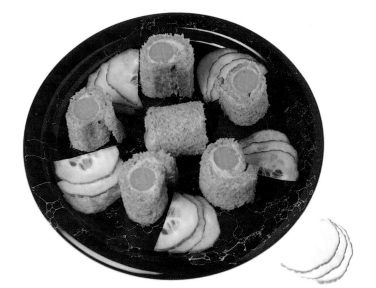

HOT DOG WHEELS

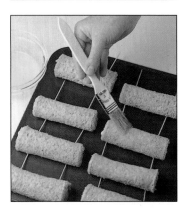
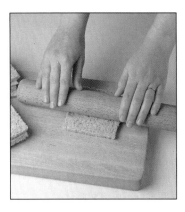
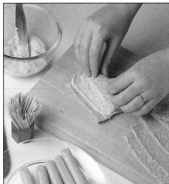

8 slices whole-wheat bread, crusts removed
1/4 cup low-fat cream cheese, softened
2 tablespoons ketchup
8 hot dogs
2 tablespoons butter, melted
Cucumber slices, to garnish

Preheat oven to 375F (190C). With a rolling pin, flatten slices of bread.

Mix cheese and ketchup together, then spread over each slice of bread. Place a hot dog at one end of bread, then roll up and secure in position with 2 wooden picks.

Place on a baking sheet. Brush with melted butter. Bake 15 minutes, until crisp. Remove picks and cut each roll into 3 pieces. Serve garnished with cucumber slices.

Makes 24 pieces.

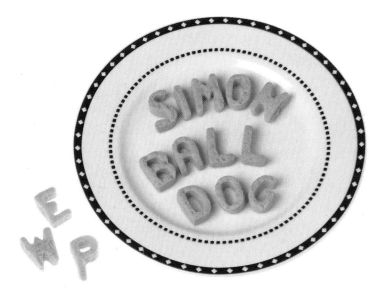

ALPHABET COOKIES

3 tablespoons smooth peanut butter
1/4 cup margarine, softened
1/4 cup light brown sugar
1 egg, beaten
1-1/2 cups all-purpose flour

Preheat oven to 350F (175C). Grease 2 or 3 baking sheets. Into a bowl, put peanut butter and margarine. Add sugar and beat until creamy.

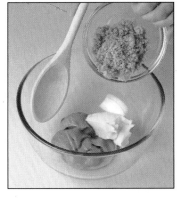

Beat in egg, then sift in the flour. Mix together to form a dough. Turn dough out onto a floured surface and knead lightly.

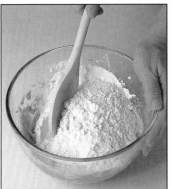

Roll out dough to about 1/4 inch thick. Using small alphabet cutters, cut out letters, then place them on prepared baking sheets. Gather up trimmings and reroll, then cut out as many letters as possible. Bake cookies 10 to 12 minutes, until lightly browned around edges. Cool on a wire rack.

Makes about 100 small letters.

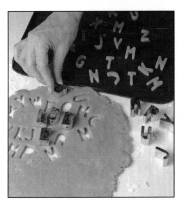

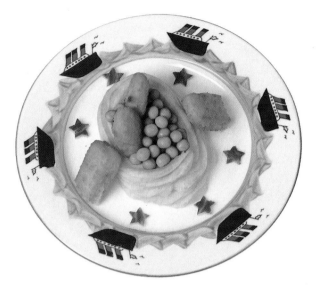

POTATO RAFTS

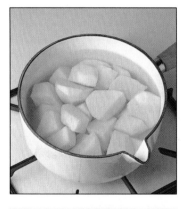

1 pound potatoes, peeled
Salt
2 tablespoons butter or margarine
1/2 cup frozen green peas
8 fish sticks
Cucumber stars, to garnish (optional)

With a sharp knife, cut potatoes into even-size pieces. In a pan of boiling lightly salted water, boil potatoes until tender. Grease a baking sheet.

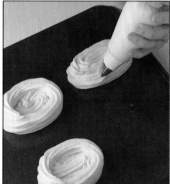

Drain potatoes. Return to pan and dry over low heat a few moments. Meanwhile, pre-heat broiler. Add butter to potatoes and mash until very smooth. Spoon into a pastry bag fitted with a large star tip and pipe 4 boat-shaped nests onto baking sheet.

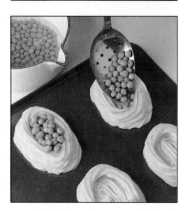

Broil potato boats until golden. Broil fish sticks until browned and cooked through. Cook peas according to package directions. To assemble, fill potato boats with peas. Halve fish sticks and place 2 halves in the center of each boat to resemble sails. Place remaining fish sticks on sides for oars.

Makes 4 servings.

Variation: Replace peas with baked beans and fish sticks with cooked sausages.

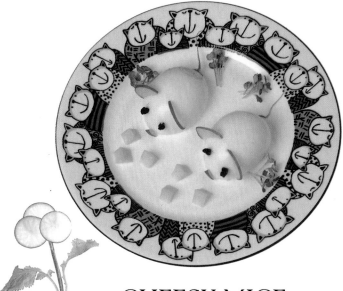

CHEESY MICE

4 eggs, hard-cooked
1/4 cup finely grated Cheddar cheese (1 ounce)
2 tablespoons low-fat cream cheese
8 radishes
16 dried currants
2 ounces Edam cheese, cut into small chunks
Radish or mustard sprouts, to garnish

With a sharp knife, carefully halve eggs lengthwise and scoop out the yolks. Put yolks into a small bowl.

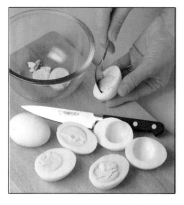

Add cheeses. Mix together until smooth. Spoon into egg whites and smooth the surface.

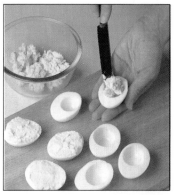

Place filled egg halves upside down. To assemble each mouse, cut slits at the pointed end of eggs, then insert small slices of radish for ears, currants for eyes and small pieces of radish for noses. Attach the radish roots for tails. To serve place 2 mice on each plate. Arrange small chunks of cheese in front of mice. Garnish with sprouts.

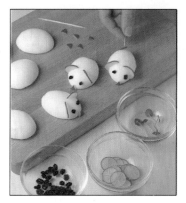

Makes 4 servings.

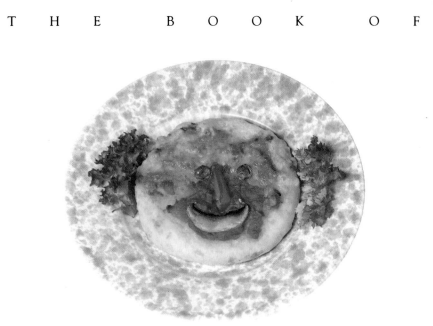

FUNNY FACE PIZZAS

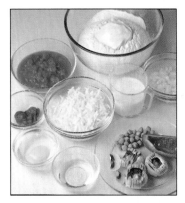

2 teaspoons vegetable oil
1/2 small onion
1 (7-oz.) can chopped tomatoes
1 tablespoon tomato paste
3 cups self-rising flour
1/3 cup margarine, chilled
1 cup shredded mild Cheddar cheese (4 ounces)
1 egg
2/3 cup milk
24 green peas
3 large button mushrooms
Red, orange or yellow bell pepper
Leaf lettuce, to garnish

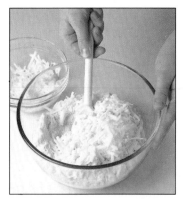

In a small saucepan, heat oil. Add onion and cook until softened. Stir in tomatoes and tomato paste; cook over medium heat 10 minutes, until thickened. Preheat oven to 400F (205C). Grease 2 baking sheets. Into a bowl, sift flour. Cut in margarine until mixture resembles bread crumbs, then stir in half the cheese. Beat egg with milk. Add to bowl and mix to form a smooth ball of dough. Divide dough into 12 pieces. Roll out each piece to a 3-inch circle. Place 6 on each baking sheet.

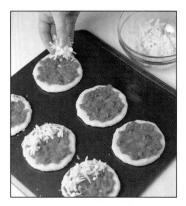

Spread tomato sauce over each dough circle. Place remaining cheese on one edge of each pizza for hair. Add peas to resemble eyes. Slice mushrooms, discarding stems. Place a slice on each pizza for the mouth. Cut bell pepper into strips and arrange on each pizza to look like a nose. Bake pizzas 12 to 15 minutes, until the edges are golden. Garnish with lettuce.

Makes 12 servings.

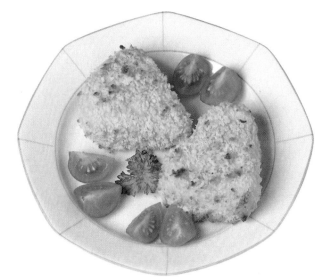

——— SURPRISE TRIANGLES ———

About 1/2 cup cooked mashed potato
6 processed cheese triangles
1 egg, beaten
1 cup fresh bread crumbs
1/4 cup peanuts, very finely chopped
12 cherry tomatoes, cut into wedges
Parsley sprigs

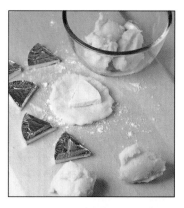

Preheat oven to 400F (205C). Grease a baking sheet. On a floured surface, spread out 1 heaped tablespoon of the potato to about 1/4 inch thick. Place a cheese triangle in the center.

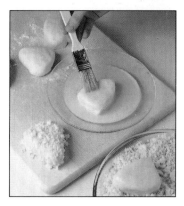

Mold the potato around the cheese, keeping a neat triangular shape. Repeat with remaining potato and cheese.

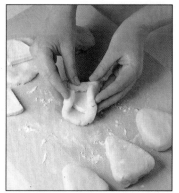

Into a shallow dish, place beaten egg. In another shallow dish, place bread crumbs and peanuts; mix together well. Dip each potato triangle in beaten egg, coating well, then coat in bread crumb mixture. Place coated potato triangles on baking sheet. Bake 15 minutes, until crisp. Serve with cherry tomatoes and garnish with parsley sprigs.

Makes 6 servings.

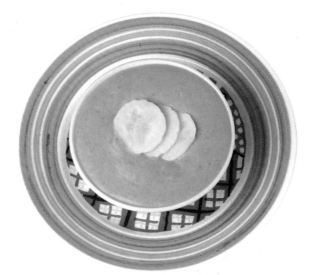

—CHOCOLATE-BANANA WHIP—

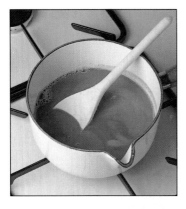

1-1/4 cups milk
1/3 cup semisweet chocolate pieces
3 tablespoons cornstarch
2 tablespoons sugar
3 small bananas
2/3 cup whipping cream

In a small saucepan, put all but 2 tablespoons of the milk and all the chocolate pieces. Place over low heat, and stir with a wooden spoon until chocolate melts.

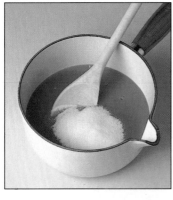

Into a bowl, put cornstarch and reserved milk and blend together. Beat in chocolate mixture. Return to saucepan, add sugar and bring to a boil, stirring. Reduce heat and cook 1 minute, stirring, until thickened. Remove from heat. Pour into a bowl and cover with a piece of plastic wrap. Refrigerate until chilled.

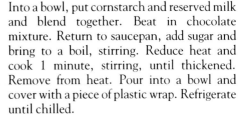

Mash 2 of the bananas. Fold mashed bananas into cool chocolate custard. In a small bowl, whip cream until soft peaks form, then fold into chocolate-banana mixture. Spoon into serving dishes and refrigerate until needed. Decorate with slices of remaining banana just before serving. (This dessert is best eaten on the day it is made.)

Makes 4 to 6 servings.

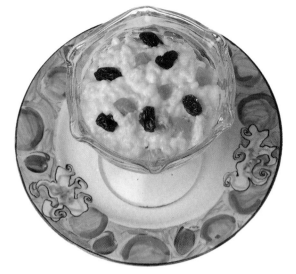

SPECIAL RICE PUDDING

1/4 cup short-grain rice
2-1/2 cups milk
2 tablespoons sugar
1 teaspoon vanilla extract
1/2 cup chopped dried apricots
1/4 cup plain or apricot-flavored yogurt
1 tablespoon each raisins and chopped apricots, to
    decorate

Into a medium-size saucepan, put rice and milk. Slowly bring to a boil. Reduce heat, cover and simmer 40 minutes, stirring occasionally.

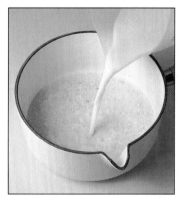

Stir in sugar, vanilla and the 1/2 cup apricots, then spoon mixture into a bowl and cool.

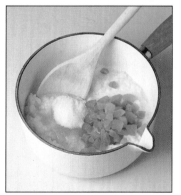

Fold in yogurt, then chill until served. To serve, spoon into serving dishes and decorate with raisins and chopped apricots.

Makes 4 to 6 servings.

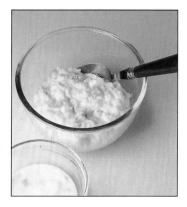

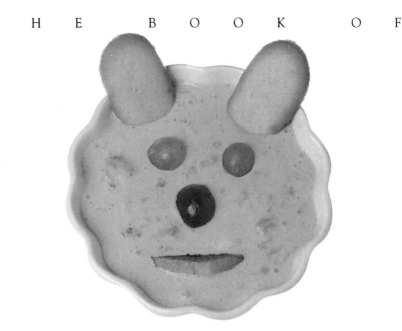

── TEDDY BEAR PUDDINGS ──

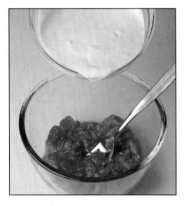

1/2 pound strawberries, rinsed and hulled
1-1/4 cups thick plain yogurt
1 tablespoon honey
8 thin oval cookies
8 seedless grapes
2 candied cherries, halved
2 slices kiwifruit, halved

In a bowl, mash the strawberries slightly (do not make them completely smooth).

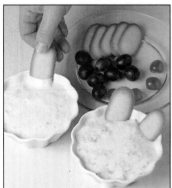

In a small bowl, whisk yogurt with honey until smooth and creamy. Add to the mashed strawberries and mix well. Divide the mixture among 4 serving dishes. Decorate by placing the cookies in position for ears.

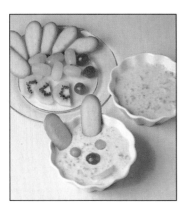

Use grapes for eyes and cherry halves for noses. Press kiwifruit halves into puddings for mouths.

Makes 4 servings.

Variations: Instead of using strawberries, cook 1 cup dried apricots until soft; puree and mix into yogurt. Or, mash 2 small, ripe bananas and add to yogurt.

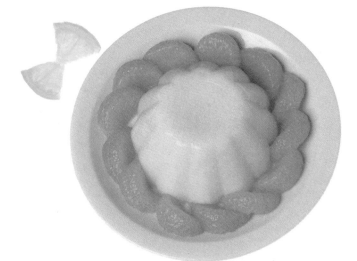

JELLY WOBBLES

4 oranges
1/4 cup sugar
2/3 cup water
5 teaspoons unflavored gelatin powder
2/3 cup plain yogurt
1 (11-oz.) can mandarin oranges in natural juice,
    drained

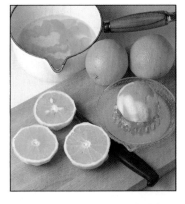

Using a vegetable peeler, pare the peel from 2 oranges and put into a saucepan with sugar and water. Bring to a boil, then simmer until the sugar has dissolved. Let stand a few minutes. Squeeze juice from all oranges and reserve.

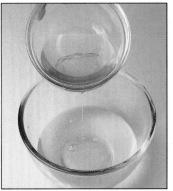

Into a medium-size bowl, strain sugar syrup, discarding orange peel. Into a small heatproof bowl, measure 3 tablespoons cold water. Sprinkle with gelatin; let stand 5 minutes to soften. Stand bowl in a pan of simmering water until gelatin dissolves. Add to strained liquid. Cool, then add orange juice and refrigerate until beginning to set.

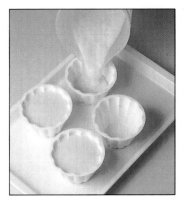

Beat in yogurt and pour into 4 or 5 small molds. Return to refrigerator 2 to 3 hours, until set. To release desserts from molds, dip each mold briefly in hot water and turn out into small dishes. Decorate with mandarin oranges.

Makes 4 to 5 servings.

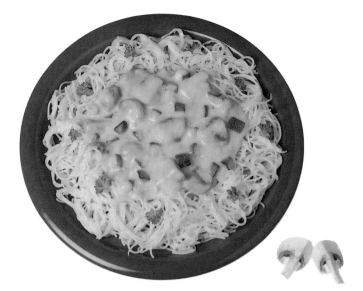

VERMICELLI NESTS

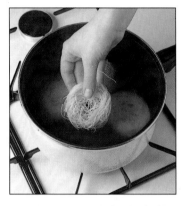

4 ounces vermicelli
2 tablespoons butter
1/3 cup chopped onion
1 zucchini, diced
6 ounces button mushrooms, quartered
2 tablespoons all-purpose flour
1 cup milk
Pinch of grated nutmeg
Salt and pepper
1/2 cup shredded Cheddar cheese (2 ounces)
Chopped fresh parsley, to garnish

Cook vermicelli in boiling salted water according to package directions until just tender to the bite.

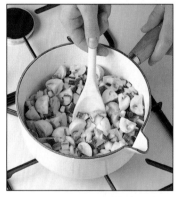

Meanwhile, in a medium-size saucepan, melt butter. Add onion, zucchini and mushrooms and cook 3 to 4 minutes, until softened. Stir in flour and cook 2 minutes longer, stirring.

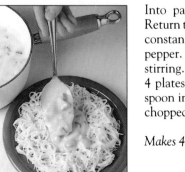

Into pan off heat, gradually stir in milk. Return to heat and simmer 2 minutes, stirring constantly. Season with nutmeg, salt and pepper. Stir in cheese and cook until melted, stirring. Drain vermicelli and divide among 4 plates. Make a hollow in the centers and spoon in vegetable sauce. Garnish with fresh chopped parsley and serve hot.

Makes 4 servings.

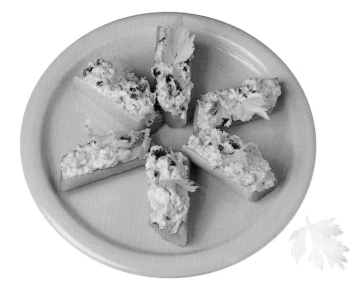

——NUTTY CELERY BOATS——

1/2 head celery, separated into stalks
1/2 cup low-fat cream cheese (4 ounces)
1/2 cup finely grated Cheddar cheese (2 ounces)
3 tablespoons crunchy peanut butter
1/4 cup raisins, chopped
1/3 cup chopped peanuts
2 tablespoons plain yogurt
Celery leaves, to garnish

Rinse celery. With a sharp knife, cut into 2-inch pieces.

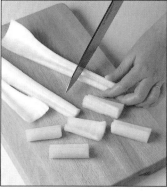

In a small bowl, combine all remaining ingredients, except celery leaves, and beat together until well blended.

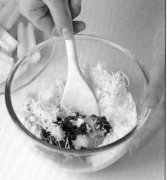

Spread filling into the celery pieces, mounding it up slightly. Garnish with celery leaves.

Makes 4 servings.

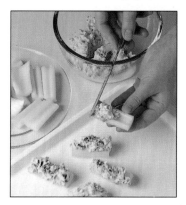

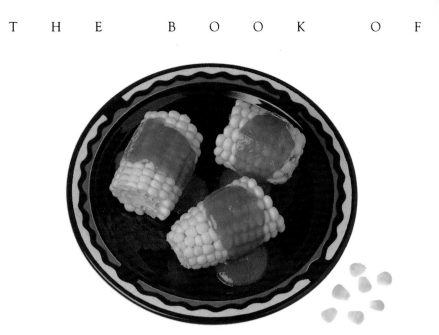

—DEVILED CORN-ON-THE-COB—

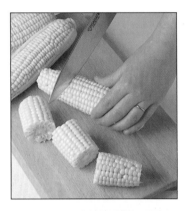

4 ears of corn
1/3 cup butter, softened
3 tablespoons ketchup
2 teaspoons Worcestershire sauce

Remove the husks and silks from corn. With a sturdy knife, cut each cob into 3 pieces. In a large saucepan of boiling water, cook corn 6 to 8 minutes, until tender.

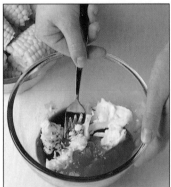

Meanwhile, preheat broiler. In a small bowl, stir together butter, ketchup and Worcestershire sauce.

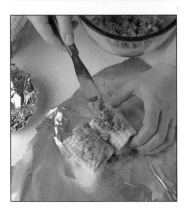

Drain corn. Spread each piece of corn with butter mixture. Put 2 pieces onto a piece of foil and wrap into a tight package; repeat with remaining corn. Place under hot broiler 5 minutes. To serve, lift the corn onto a plate and top with deviled butter from foil.

Makes 4 to 6 servings.

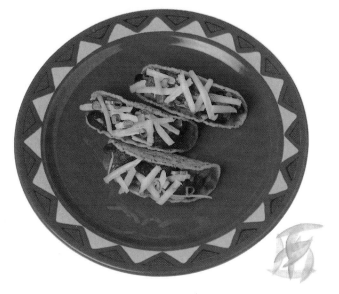

MINI TACOS

1 tablespoon vegetable oil
1 small onion, finely chopped
3 tomatoes, peeled and diced
1/2 green bell pepper, chopped
1 tablespoon tomato paste
1/2 teaspoon chili sauce (optional)
1 (7-oz.) can red kidney beans, rinsed and drained
12 mini taco shells
1/2 cup shredded Cheddar cheese (2 ounces)
3 green onions, chopped

Preheat oven to 350F (175C). In a medium-size saucepan, heat oil. Add onion and cook until softened, stirring occasionally.

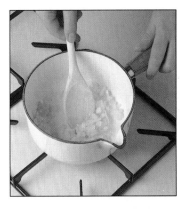

Add tomatoes, bell pepper, tomato paste, chili sauce (if using) and kidney beans. Simmer 7 to 8 minutes, until vegetables are softened.

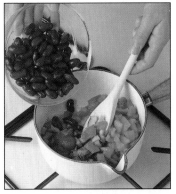

Meanwhile, put taco shells onto a baking sheet and warm 3 to 4 minutes. Divide filling among taco shells, then top with cheese and a little chopped green onions.

Makes 3 to 4 servings.

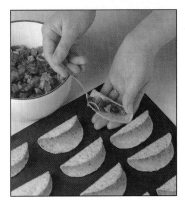

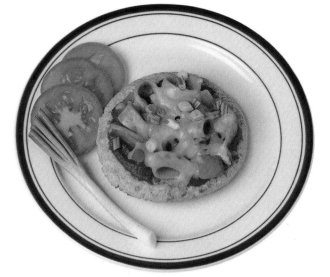

PITA PIZZAS

4 small whole-wheat pita breads
Margarine, softened
4 teaspoons tomato paste
2 large tomatoes, chopped
4 large slices salami or cooked ham
Pinch of Italian seasoning
1/2 cup shredded Cheddar cheese (2 ounces)
3 green onions, chopped
Green onions and sliced tomatoes, to serve

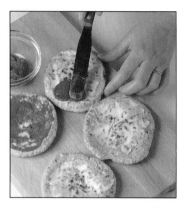

Preheat broiler. Spread a little margarine over one side of each pita bread. Spread 1 teaspoon tomato paste on top of each.

Divide chopped tomatoes among pitas. Cut salami slices into strips, then arrange on top. Sprinkle with Italian seasoning.

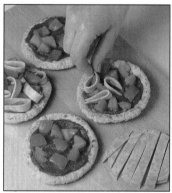

Sprinkle with cheese and green onions. Place under hot broiler 3 to 5 minutes, until heated through and cheese has melted. Serve with green onions and sliced tomatoes.

Makes 4 servings.

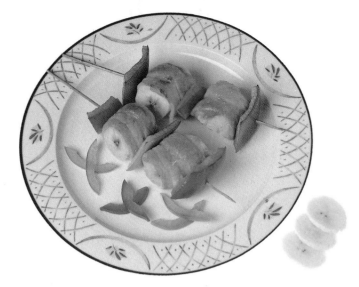

— BANANA & BACON KABOBS —

4 large bananas (slightly under-ripe)
8 very lean bacon slices, halved
1 red bell pepper, cut into pieces
1 green bell pepper, cut into pieces
1 tablespoon vegetable oil
1 tablespoon soy sauce
1 teaspoon honey
Bell pepper strips, to garnish

Preheat broiler. Peel bananas, then cut each crosswise into 4 pieces. Wrap each piece of banana in a halved bacon slice.

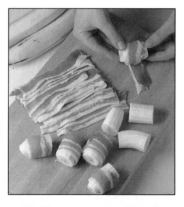

Thread bacon rolls onto bamboo skewers alternately with bell peppers.

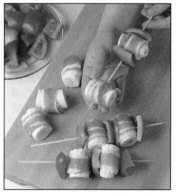

In a small bowl, mix oil, soy sauce and honey together. Brush over kabobs. Place under hot broiler, turning them during cooking and brushing them with oil mixture, until bacon is golden and crisp. Serve hot garnished with bell pepper strips.

Makes 4 servings.

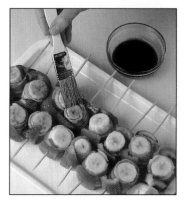

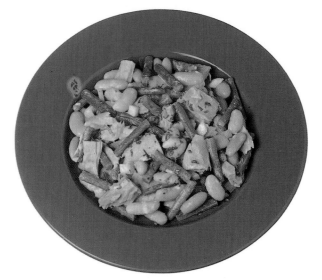

—— TUNA & BEAN SALAD ——

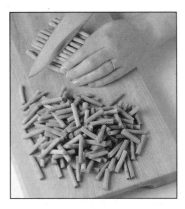

6 ounces small green beans
1 tablespoon finely chopped onion
1 (14-oz.) can cannellini beans, drained
1 (7-oz.) can tuna in water, drained
3 tablespoons low-fat plain yogurt
1 tablespoon lemon juice
1 tablespoon olive oil
Salt and pepper
Shredded lettuce, to serve (optional)
Chopped fresh parsley, to garnish

With a knife, trim beans and cut into 1-inch pieces. Put into a pan of boiling water and cook 3 to 4 minutes, until crisp-tender.

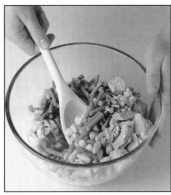

Drain beans and rinse under cold water to cool. In a medium-size bowl, combine green beans with onion, cannellini beans and tuna. Mix together, breaking up tuna.

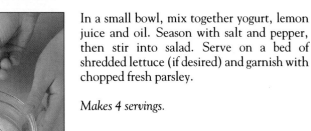

In a small bowl, mix together yogurt, lemon juice and oil. Season with salt and pepper, then stir into salad. Serve on a bed of shredded lettuce (if desired) and garnish with chopped fresh parsley.

Makes 4 servings.

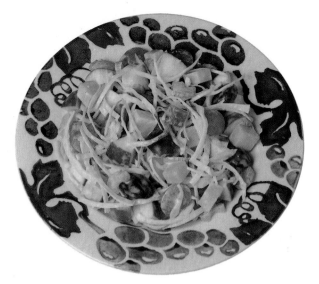

— FRUITY CHEESE COLESLAW —

1 red apple
1 tablespoon lemon juice
2 cups finely shredded white cabbage
2 celery stalks, finely sliced
4 ounces seedless green grapes
4 ounces seedless black grapes
2 ounces Cheddar cheese
2 ounces Gouda cheese
2 tablespoons vegetable oil
2 tablespoons plain yogurt
1 teaspoon honey

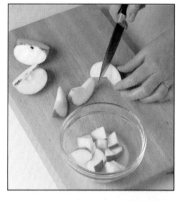

With a knife, core apple, then cut into small chunks. Toss in lemon juice to prevent browning.

Remove apple from juice (reserving juice). In a medium-size bowl, combine apple, cabbage, celery and grapes. Cut cheeses into small cubes, then add to other ingredients.

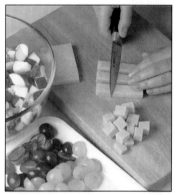

In a small bowl, mix together reserved lemon juice, oil, yogurt and honey. Beat until smooth, then fold into salad ingredients.

Makes 4 to 6 servings.

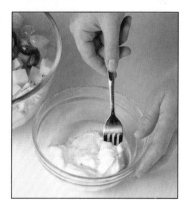

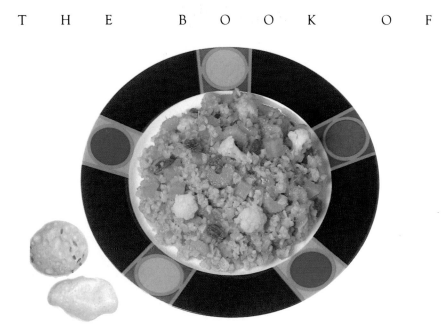

—SPICY VEGETABLE BULGUR—

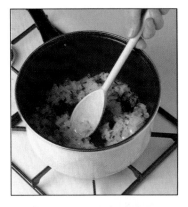

2 tablespoons vegetable oil
1 onion, chopped
1 cup bulgur wheat
1 tablespoon mild curry powder
2 carrots, diced
2 celery stalks, chopped
1-3/4 cups cauliflowerets
2-1/2 cups hot vegetable stock
1/4 cup dark raisins or golden raisins
2 tablespoons fruit chutney
Salt and pepper

In a large saucepan, heat half the oil. Add onion and cook until softened, stirring occasionally.

Add remaining oil, then stir in bulgur wheat and curry powder. Cook over low heat 1 minute. Add prepared vegetables, then pour in stock. Cover and simmer 15 minutes, until vegetables are tender.

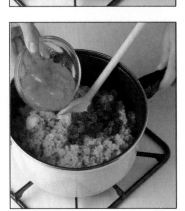

Stir in raisins and chutney. Season to taste and heat through. Serve with small poppadums (crisp Indian wafers).

Makes 4 servings.

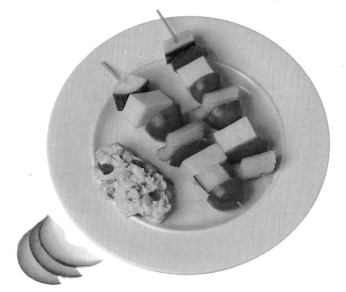

SALAD KABOBS

2 celery stalks
4-inch piece cucumber
6 ounces Gouda or Edam cheese, cubed
1 red bell pepper, cut into pieces
8 cherry tomatoes, halved
DIP:
2 tablespoons low-fat cream cheese, softened
1 ripe avocado
1 tomato, peeled and finely chopped
3 green onions, finely chopped
Salt and pepper

With a knife, cut celery and cucumber into 1/2- to 1-inch pieces.

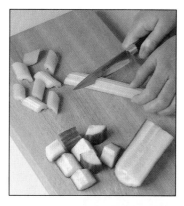

Thread celery and cucumber onto 8 small bamboo skewers alternately with cheese, bell pepper and tomato halves.

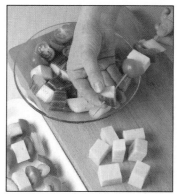

Into a small bowl, put cream cheese. With a knife, cut avocado in half and scoop out flesh. Add to cheese and mash together well. Stir in chopped tomato and green onions. Season with salt and pepper. Serve as a dip with kabobs.

Makes 4 servings.

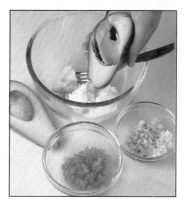

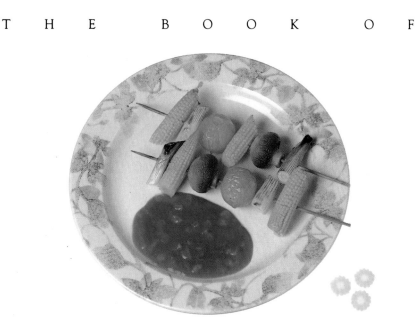

─── VEGETABLE KABOBS ───

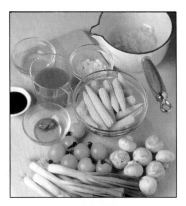

1 bunch large green onions, trimmed
1 (15-oz.) can baby corn, drained
8 cherry tomatoes
1/4 pound button mushrooms, trimmed
Vegetable oil for brushing
BARBECUE SAUCE:
1 tablespoon vegetable oil
1 tablespoon finely chopped onion
2 teaspoons all-purpose flour
2/3 cup tomato juice
2 teaspoons wine vinegar
2 teaspoons Worcestershire sauce
1 teaspoon honey
1/2 teaspoon mustard powder

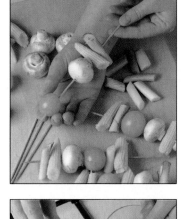

Preheat broiler. With a knife, cut green onions into 1-inch pieces; halve baby corn crosswise, if large. Arrange a selection of all vegetables on 8 small bamboo skewers. Brush vegetables with oil and cook under hot broiler 5 to 8 minutes, turning halfway through cooking time.

Meanwhile, make sauce. In a small saucepan, heat oil. Add onion and cook, stirring, 2 to 3 minutes, until softened. Stir in flour, then add tomato juice and remaining ingredients. Cook 3 minutes, stirring constantly, until thickened. Serve with kabobs.

Makes 8.

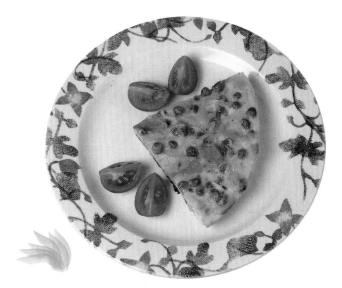

SPANISH OMELET

1 tablespoon olive oil
1/2 onion, finely chopped
4 bacon slices, chopped
1/2 orange, red or green bell pepper, cut into thin strips
1 heaped cup grated potatoes
4 eggs, beaten
Salt and pepper
1/3 cup frozen green peas, thawed
2 tomatoes, cut into wedges, to serve

In a medium-size nonstick skillet, heat oil. Add onion and bacon and cook 2 to 3 minutes, stirring, until onion is lightly golden. Discard some of the fat. Meanwhile, preheat broiler.

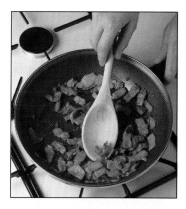

Add bell pepper and potatoes to skillet and continue cooking 4 to 5 minutes, stirring occasionally, until potato softens.

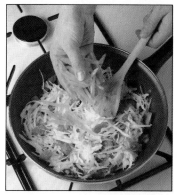

In a small bowl, beat eggs together with salt and pepper. Pour into skillet, then add peas. Continue cooking over medium heat 5 to 10 minutes, until eggs are set. Place skillet under broiler 1 minute to set top of omelet. Turn out omelet, cut into 4 wedges and serve hot, garnished with tomato wedges.

Makes 4 servings.

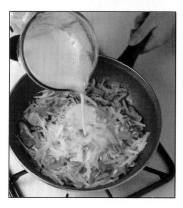

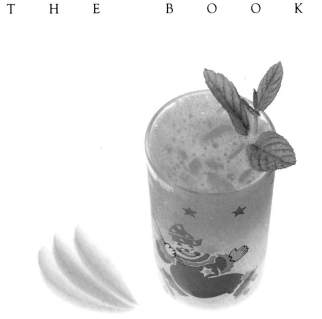

APPLE ZING

2 ripe pears, peeled and cored
2 cups apple juice
Crushed ice
2-1/2 cups chilled ginger ale
Apple slices or mint sprigs, to decorate

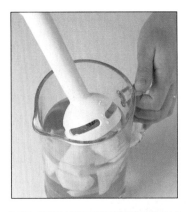

Use a hand blender or food processor to blend the pears and apple juice until smooth.

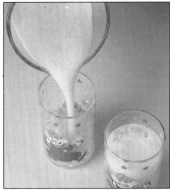

Into 4 tall glasses, spoon crushed ice. Pour apple juice mixture over ice.

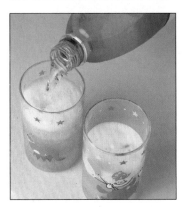

Fill glasses with ginger ale, then decorate with apple slices or mint sprigs. Serve immediately.

Makes 4 servings.

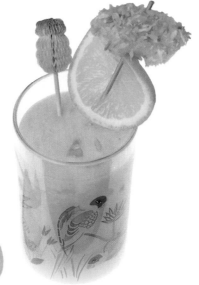

—CARIBBEAN FRUIT COCKTAIL—

6 tablespoons shredded coconut
1 (7-oz.) can pineapple slices in juice
2 ripe bananas, peeled
2 cups chilled orange juice
Crushed ice
1 small orange, sliced

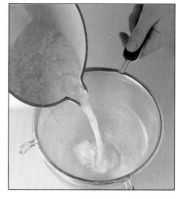

Into a small saucepan, put 4 tablespoons of the coconut and 1-1/2 cups water. Bring to a boil, then simmer 3 minutes. Cool, then strain liquid, discarding coconut.

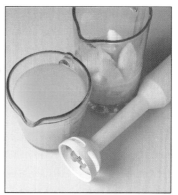

Lightly toast remaining coconut in a dry skillet over medium heat, stirring with a wooden spoon. Let cool. Reserve 2 pineapple rings for decoration. Use a hand blender or food processor to blend pineapple rings with pineapple juice, coconut liquid, bananas and orange juice until smooth.

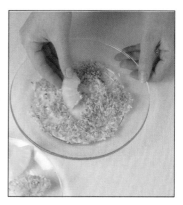

Into 4 glasses, spoon crushed ice. Pour fruit juice mixture over ice. With a knife, cut reserved pineapple rings into 4 or 5 pieces. Toss in toasted coconut. Thread pineapple pieces and orange slices onto wooden skewers or bamboo sticks and use to decorate each drink. Serve at once.

Makes 4 servings.

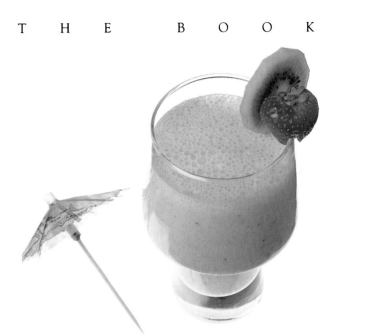

– STRAWBERRY-YOGURT WHIZZ –

1/2 pound strawberries
1-1/4 cups milk
1-1/4 cups natural or strawberry-flavored yogurt
2 scoops vanilla ice cream or frozen yogurt
1 kiwi fruit (optional), sliced

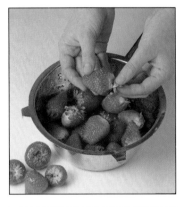

Reserve 4 strawberries for decoration; cap remaining strawberries.

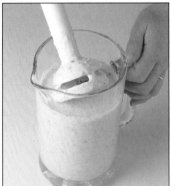

Use a hand blender or food processor to blend milk, yogurt, strawberries and ice cream until smooth.

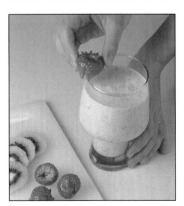

Into 3 or 4 glasses, pour strawberry drink. Decorate with reserved strawberries and slices of kiwifruit, if using.

Makes 3 or 4 servings.

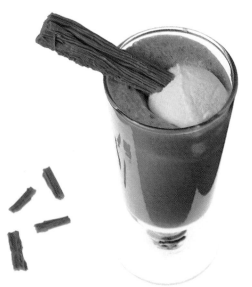

MALTED MILKSHAKES

1 (12-oz.) can evaporated milk
2 cups milk
3 tablespoons unsweetened cocoa powder
2 teaspoons light brown sugar
1/4 cup malt-flavored drink powder
8 scoops vanilla ice cream
4 chocolate candy sticks

Put 4 glass tumblers into refrigerator to chill 30 minutes.

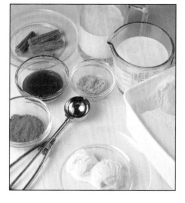

Use a hand blender or food processor to blend both milks, cocoa powder, sugar, malt-flavored drink powder and half the ice cream 2 minutes, until frothy; if necessary, do in 2 batches.

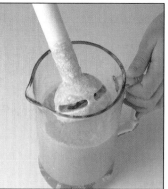

Pour malted mixture into chilled glasses. Top each drink with a scoop of ice cream and a chocolate candy stick. Serve with straws.

Makes 4 servings.

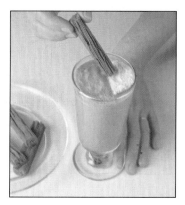

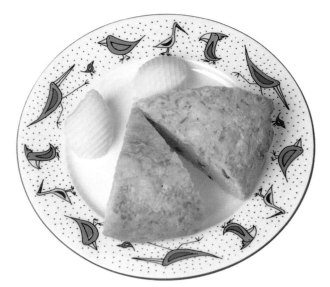

CHEESE BISCUITS

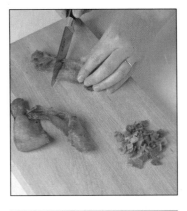

4 bacon slices
2 cups self-rising flour
1 teaspoon baking powder
1/2 teaspoon salt
1 teaspoon mustard powder
1/4 cup margarine, chilled
1/2 cup shredded Cheddar cheese (2 ounces)
1/2 cup milk, plus extra for brushing
Butter or margarine curls, to serve

Preheat broiler and oven to 425F (220C). Grease a baking sheet. Broil bacon until crisp, then cut into small pieces.

Into a bowl, sift flour, baking powder, salt and mustard. Cut in margarine, then add bacon and three-quarters of the cheese.

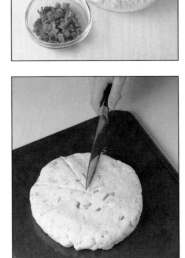

Stir in the 1/2 cup milk, then mix to form a softened dough. Knead on a lightly floured surface until smooth. With fingers, press out dough to a circle 6 inches in diameter. Place on a baking sheet and with a knife mark into 6 wedges. Brush top with a little milk, then sprinkle with remaining cheese. Bake 12 to 15 minutes, until puffed and golden. Serve warm with butter curls.

Makes 6.

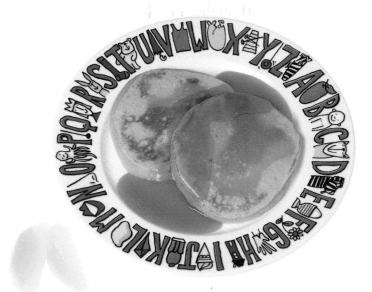

–SAUCY CORNMEAL PANCAKES–

1 cup all-purpose flour
3 tablespoons sugar
1 teaspoon baking powder
1 cup cornmeal
2 eggs
1-1/4 cups milk
2 tablespoons vegetable oil
BUTTERSCOTCH SAUCE:
3 tablespoons butter
3/4 cup light brown sugar
2 tablespoons light corn syrup
3 tablespoons half and half

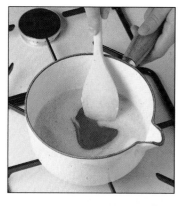

To make sauce, in a small saucepan, combine all ingredients.

Over medium heat, heat mixture until sugar dissolves, stirring constantly. Set aside. In a medium-size bowl, put flour, sugar, baking powder and cornmeal. In another bowl, beat together eggs, milk and 1 tablespoon of the oil. Add to dry ingredients and beat until smooth.

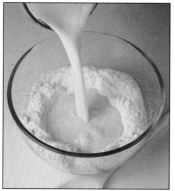

Heat a large, nonstick skillet over medium-high heat. Brush with a little of the remaining oil. Drop 2 or 3 large spoonfuls of batter onto skillet, allowing space for each pancake to spread. Cook until bubbles appear on the surface, then turn over and cook other side until golden. Repeat with remaining batter, keeping the pancakes warm until all are cooked. Serve with butterscotch sauce.

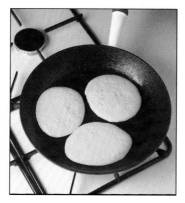

Makes 16.

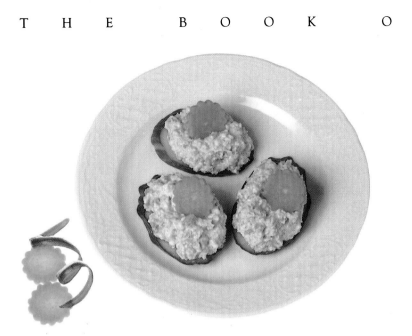

CUCUMBER SNACKS

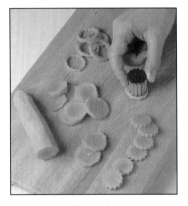

1 large carrot, peeled
2 celery stalks, trimmed
1 cup sunflower seed kernels
1/4 cup plain yogurt
2 tablespoons mayonnaise
1 cucumber

With a knife, cut 16 thin slices from carrot, then, using a small fancy cookie cutter, cut out decorations. Set aside. Coarsely chop rest of carrot and celery. Put into a food processor with carrot trimmings and process until finely chopped. Transfer to a bowl.

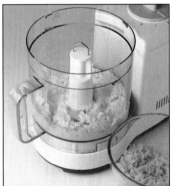

Into the food processor or blender, put sunflower kernels, yogurt and mayonnaise. Process until a paste forms. Spoon paste mixture into bowl with the chopped carrot and celery and mix together.

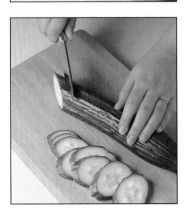

With a knife, cut 16 cucumber slices, cutting on a slant to make diagonal slices. Place a spoonful of vegetable mixture on each cucumber slice, then decorate with carrot shapes.

Makes 16.

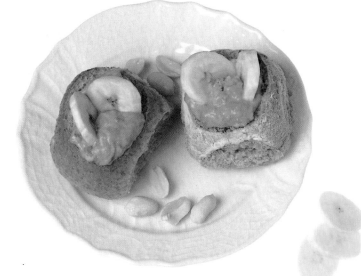

BANANA CUSHIONS

8 small whole-wheat bread rolls
2 tablespoons crunchy peanut butter
2 tablespoons cream cheese, softened
3 small bananas
Peanuts, for garnish (optional)

With a knife, cut a small slice off the top of each bread roll. With the point of knife, scoop out middle of each roll.

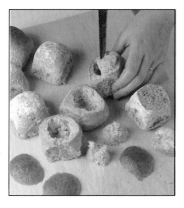

In a bowl, combine peanut butter and cream cheese, then beat together. Roughly mash 2 bananas, then fold into peanut-butter mixture. Divide among the bread rolls.

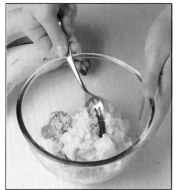

Slice remaining banana and use to decorate each roll. Serve immediately. Garnish with peanuts, if desired.

Makes 8.

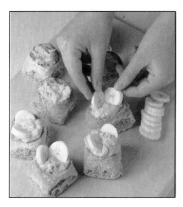

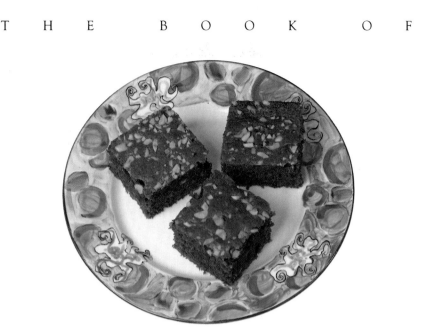

NUTTY BROWNIES

1-1/4 cups self-rising flour
1 cup packed light brown sugar
3/4 cup lightly toasted, chopped hazelnuts or pecans
1/2 cup butter
4 ounces semisweet chocolate, broken into small pieces
2 eggs, beaten
5 tablespoons milk
1 teaspoon vanilla extract

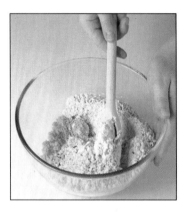

Preheat oven to 350F (175C). Grease an 8-inch square cake pan. In a medium-size bowl, put flour, sugar and three-quarters of the nuts. Mix together.

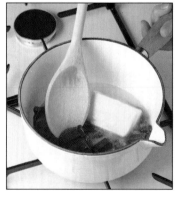

In a small saucepan, melt butter and chocolate over low heat Cool slightly.

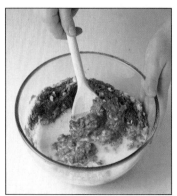

Into another bowl, put eggs, milk and vanilla and beat together. Add to flour mixture with melted butter and chocolate. Beat until combined. Pour into prepared pan, scatter nuts over top and bake 25 to 30 minutes, until firm. Cool on a wire rack, then cut into 12 pieces.

Makes 12.

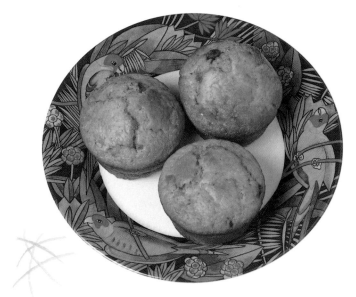

ORANGE MUFFINS

2-1/2 cups all-purpose flour
1 tablespoon baking powder
Pinch of salt
1/2 cup packed light brown sugar
Grated zest and juice of 1 orange
2 eggs
1 cup milk
1/4 cup butter, melted
1 cup semisweet chocolate pieces

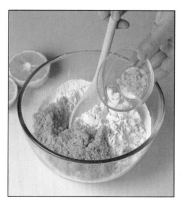

Preheat oven to 400F (205C). Grease a 12-cup muffin pan or line with paper cupcake cups. Into a medium-size bowl, sift flour, baking powder and salt. Stir in sugar and orange zest.

In another bowl, beat together orange juice, eggs, milk and butter. Pour onto dry ingredients. Add chocolate pieces and stir together just until blended. Do not overmix.

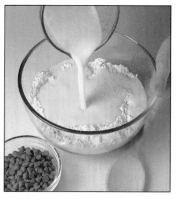

Spoon batter into muffin pan, filling each cup about two-thirds full; put water in any unfilled cups so they do not burn during baking. Bake 20 to 25 minutes, until golden-brown. Cool on a wire rack.

Makes 10 to 12.

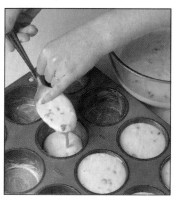

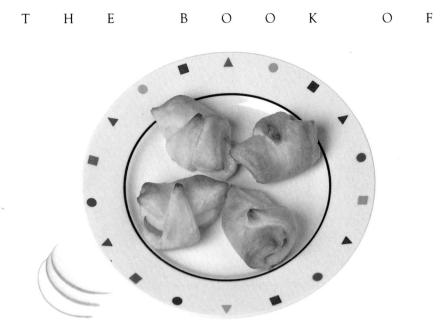

—MINI SAVORY CROISSANTS—

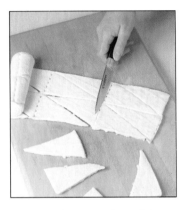

24 refrigerated ready-to-cook mini croissants
(1 package)
1/4 pound Cheddar cheese or processed cheese slices
1 small apple
2 ounces thinly sliced smoked ham
Milk, to glaze

Preheat oven to 400F (205C). Grease 2 baking sheets. Open package of croissant dough as directed on label. Unfold dough onto a board and separate the croissants along perforations.

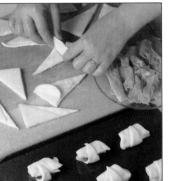

With a knife, cut cheese into 24 small triangles to fit croissants. Lay a piece of cheese on each croissant. Cut apple into 12 small slices. Place an apple slice at broad end on top of cheese on 12 of the croissants. Roll up each of these croissants toward the point, then place on baking sheet.

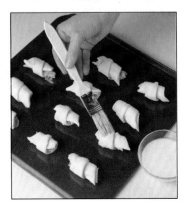

Divide ham between remaining 12 croissants. Roll up each croissant toward the point, then place on baking sheet. Brush croissants with milk. Bake in oven 10 minutes, until golden-brown. Serve warm.

Makes 24.

Variation: If mini croissants are not available, cut regular croissants in half and fill as above.

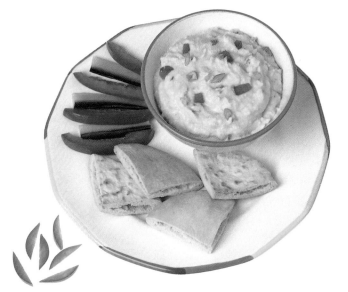

——————— VEGETABLE DIP ———————

1 (14-oz.) can garbanzo beans, drained
1 garlic clove, crushed
1/4 cup thick plain yogurt
1/2 red bell pepper, finely diced
3 green onions, finely chopped
Salt and pepper
8 small pita breads
Cucumber and red bell pepper strips, to garnish

Preheat oven to 350F (175C). Into a food processor or blender, put garbanzo beans, garlic and yogurt. Process until smooth. Transfer to a bowl.

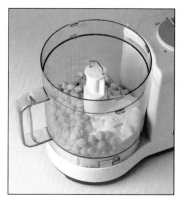

Fold in bell pepper and green onions. Season to taste with salt and pepper.

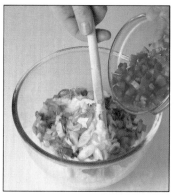

With a knife, cut pita breads into quarters. Place on a baking sheet and toast in oven about 5 minutes, until warm and crisp. Serve at once with dip. Garnish with cucumber and bell pepper strips.

Makes 4 to 6 servings.

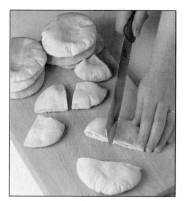

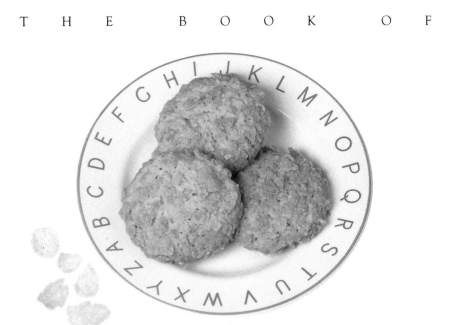

COCONUT CRISPS

2/3 cup butter or margarine, softened
1 egg
1/2 teaspoon vanilla extract
1/2 cup packed light brown sugar
1 cup shredded coconut
2/3 cup rolled oats
1 cup self-rising flour
2 cups cornflakes, lightly crushed

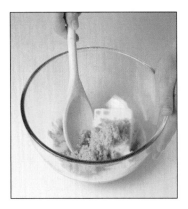

Preheat oven to 325F (165C). Grease 2 baking sheets. Into a medium-size bowl, put butter, egg, vanilla and sugar. Beat until creamy.

Stir in coconut, oats and flour, and mix to form a dough. Roll dough into about 25 balls, each the size of a large walnut.

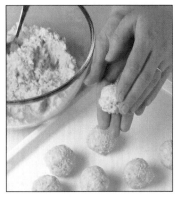

Put crushed cornflakes on a plate. Lightly press dough balls in cornflakes to coat all over. Place on baking sheets. Bake about 15 minutes, until lightly browned. Transfer to a wire rack to cool.

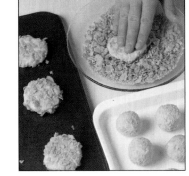

Makes about 25.

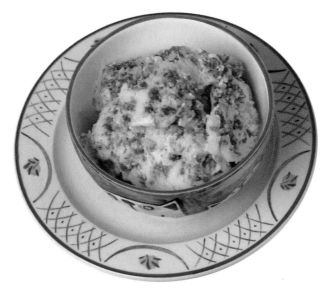

—BROWN BREAD ICE CREAM—

1-1/4 cups milk
1/3 cup granulated sugar
4 egg yolks
1 teaspoon vanilla extract
1-1/2 cups whole-wheat bread crumbs
1/2 cup packed dark brown sugar

In a saucepan, heat milk almost to a simmer. In a bowl, put granulated sugar and egg yolks and beat together. Stir hot milk into sugar mixture. Return to saucepan. Cook over very low heat, stirring, until thickened. Let cool.

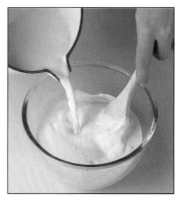

Stir vanilla into custard. Pour into a shallow freezerproof bowl and freeze until crystals form around edge of mixture. Turn out ice cream into a bowl and beat until smooth. Return to freezerproof bowl and freeze again.

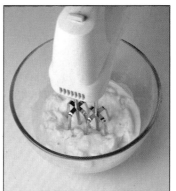

Meanwhile, preheat oven to 400F (205C). In a bowl, combine bread crumbs and brown sugar. Spread out on a nonstick baking sheet. Bake until crumbs are golden-brown, stirring occasionally with a long-handled wooden spoon to give an even color. Let cool. Stir into ice cream. Freeze until 15 minutes before serving, then transfer to refrigerator to soften slightly.

Makes 4 to 6 servings.

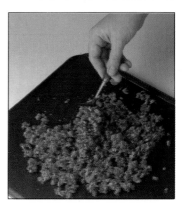

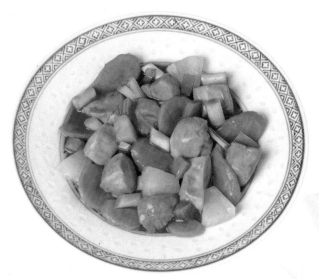

— SWEET & SOUR CHICKEN —

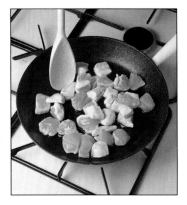

3/4 pound skinless, boneless chicken thighs, cut into
   bite-size pieces
2 tablespoons vegetable oil
1 large carrot, thinly sliced
1/2 green bell pepper, diced
2 canned pineapple rings, drained and chopped
4 green onions, chopped
2 tablespoons white-wine vinegar
2 tablespoons soy sauce
2 tablespoons ketchup
2 tablespoons honey
2 teaspoons cornstarch
3 tablespoons pineapple juice

In a medium-size skillet, fry chicken in oil 6 to 8 minutes.

Add carrot and bell pepper, then cook 3 minutes longer. Stir in pineapple and green onions. In a small bowl, combine vinegar, soy sauce, ketchup and honey, then pour into skillet. Bring to a boil, then reduce heat and simmer 4 to 5 minutes.

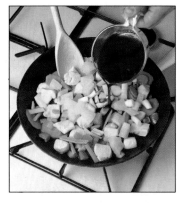

In a small bowl, blend cornstarch with pineapple juice. Stir into skillet and continue cooking, stirring, until thickened. Serve with rice or noodles.

Makes 3 to 4 servings.

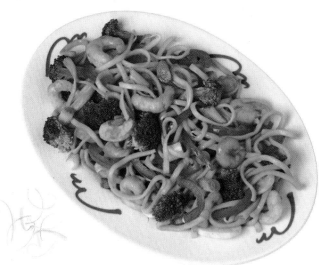

CHOP SUEY SALAD

1/4 pound Chinese egg noodles
1 cup small broccoli flowerets
1/2 pound bean sprouts
2/3 cup thinly sliced mushrooms
5 green onions, chopped
1/2 red and 1/2 green or yellow bell peppers, cut into
   thin slivers
1/4 pound cooked shelled shrimp
3 tablespoons vegetable oil
1 tablespoon soy sauce
Pinch of ground ginger

Break the noodles into small pieces. In a pan of boiling water, cook noodles 3 to 4 minutes, until tender. Drain and cool.

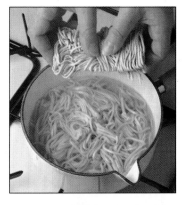

With a knife, cut broccoli flowerets into small pieces. In a pan of boiling water, blanch 3 minutes. Drain and rinse in cold water, then drain again. Rinse bean sprouts. In a bowl, combine bean sprouts, mushrooms, green onions, bell peppers, shrimp, broccoli and noodles.

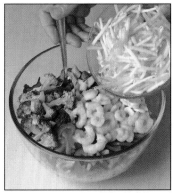

In a small bowl, combine oil, soy sauce and ginger. Beat until well blended. Pour dressing over salad and toss so all ingredients are coated. Cover with plastic wrap and chill until ready to serve.

Makes 4 servings.

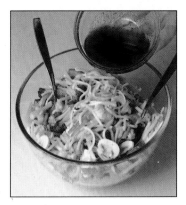

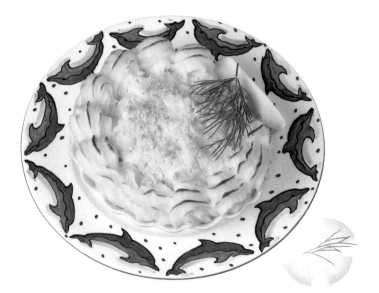

──── FISH IN POTATO NESTS ────

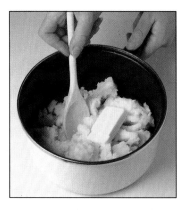

1-1/2 pounds potatoes
3 tablespoons milk
1/4 cup butter or margarine
1/2 pound cod or haddock fillet
1-1/4 cups milk
2 tablespoons all-purpose flour
Salt and pepper
2 hard-cooked eggs, chopped
2 tablespoons fresh bread crumbs
Fresh dill sprigs, to garnish

In a saucepan of boiling lightly salted water, cook potatoes until tender. Drain, return to pan and mash. Add the 3 tablespoons milk and half the butter; beat until smooth.

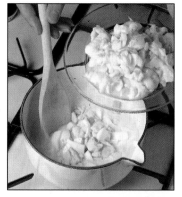

Into another pan, put fish and milk. Cover and poach 6 to 7 minutes, until the fish just begins to flake. Remove fish and reserve milk to make sauce. Into a bowl, flake fish, discarding skin and any bones. In a pan, melt remaining butter. Stir in flour, then cook 1 minute, stirring. Off heat, gradually stir in reserved poaching milk. Simmer 1 to 2 minutes, stirring, until thick and smooth. Fold in fish, salt, pepper and eggs. Preheat broiler.

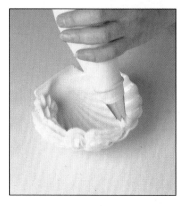

Put mashed potato into a pastry bag fitted with a 1-inch star tip. Pipe a border around edge of 4 shallow heatproof dishes or shells. Spoon fish mixture into dishes, then scatter bread crumbs over top. Place under hot broiler until golden-brown and warmed through. Serve garnished with dill.

Makes 4 servings.

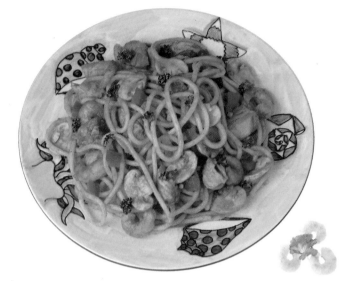

SPAGHETTI MARINARA

1/2 pound spaghetti
1 tablespoon olive oil
1 small onion, finely chopped
1 garlic clove, crushed
1-1/2 cups sliced button mushrooms
1/2 red or green bell pepper, diced
1-1/4 cups chopped canned tomatoes, sieved, with
    some liquid drained off
1 (7-oz.) can pink salmon, drained
1/4 pound cooked shelled shrimp
Pinch of dried leaf oregano
Salt and pepper

Cook pasta in boiling salted water according to package directions. Drain well.

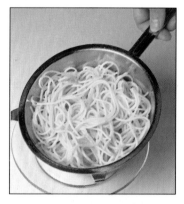

Meanwhile, in a saucepan, heat oil. Add onion, garlic, mushrooms and bell pepper and cook 3 to 4 minutes, until onion is softened. Add tomatoes and simmer 2 to 3 minutes longer. Remove any salmon bones and skin, then flake. Add to sauce with shrimp, oregano, salt and pepper.

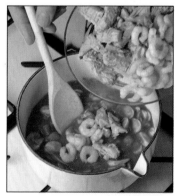

Return drained spaghetti to pan and mix together with sauce. Heat through before serving.

Makes 4 servings.

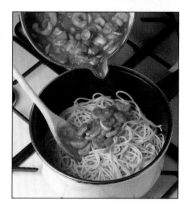

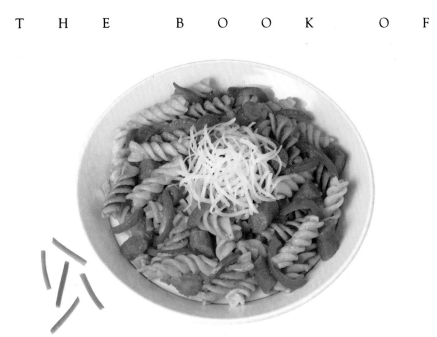

SALAMI PASTA

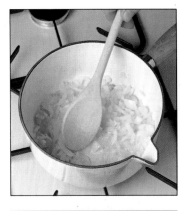

2 tablespoons olive oil
1 onion, finely chopped
1 garlic clove, crushed
1 red bell pepper, finely sliced
1 (14-oz.) can chopped tomatoes
1/2 teaspoon sugar
1/2 teaspoon dried leaf oregano
Salt and pepper
4 cups pasta shapes
1/4 pound salami stick, sliced
1/2 cup shredded Cheddar cheese (2 ounces)

In a medium-size saucepan, heat oil. Add onion and cook over medium heat 3 to 4 minutes, until softened.

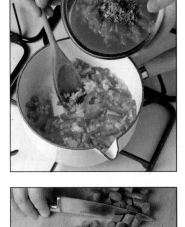

Add garlic and bell pepper, and cook a few minutes longer. Stir in tomatoes, sugar, oregano, salt and pepper. Cover and simmer 10 minutes, stirring occasionally.

Meanwhile, cook pasta in boiling salted water according to package directions just until tender to the bite. Drain well, then return to saucepan. Stir in salami and tomato sauce, then heat through. Serve sprinkled with cheese.

Makes 4 servings.

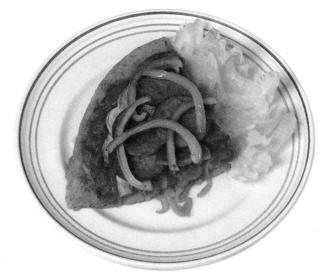

POTATO PIZZA

1 pound potatoes, peeled
2 tablespoons butter or margarine
1/4 cup whole-wheat flour
Salt
TOPPING:
1 tablespoon olive oil
1 small onion, sliced
1 (7-oz.) can chopped tomatoes
1 tablespoon tomato paste
1/2 teaspoon dried leaf basil
2/3 cup sliced mushrooms
2 ounces sliced pepperoni
1/2 green bell pepper, cut into thin strips
Lettuce leaves, to serve (optional)

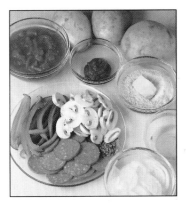

Preheat oven to 400F (205C). Grease a baking sheet. With a knife, cut potatoes into even-size pieces. In pan of lightly salted, boiling water, cook potatoes until tender. Drain well, then return to pan and mash. Beat in butter and flour, then season with salt. Mix to make a dough. Turn out dough onto baking sheet and with your fingers spread out to an 8-inch circle. Bake about 10 minutes, until the edge of pizza begins to crisp.

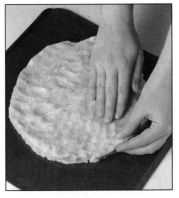

Meanwhile, in a small saucepan, heat oil. Add onion and cook over medium heat 2 to 3 minutes, until softened. Stir in tomatoes, tomato paste and basil, then simmer 5 minutes longer, until thickened. Spread sauce over potato base. Arrange mushrooms over sauce, then pepperoni. Place strips of bell pepper in a crisscross pattern over the pizza. Bake 20 minutes. Serve hot, cut into wedges. Serve with lettuce leaves, if desired.

Makes 3 to 4 servings.

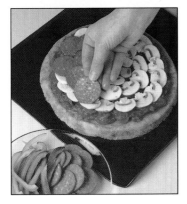

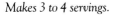

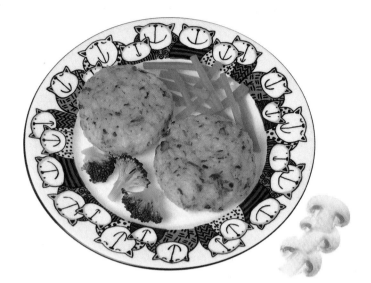

—MUSHROOM & RICE PATTIES—

1-1/4 cups long-grain rice
1 tablespoon vegetable oil
1/3 cup very finely chopped onion
2-1/2 cups finely chopped mushrooms (6.ounces)
1/2 cup shredded Cheddar cheese (2 ounces)
Salt and pepper
All-purpose flour
Cooked vegetables, to serve

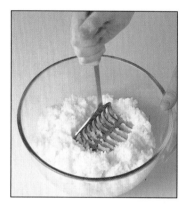

Cook rice according to package directions until very tender. Drain well if necessary, then put rice into a bowl. Mash to break up grains. Preheat oven to 400F (205C). Grease a baking sheet.

In a medium-size saucepan, heat oil. Add onion and mushrooms and cook until all liquid has evaporated from mushrooms. Stir into rice with cheese, salt and pepper.

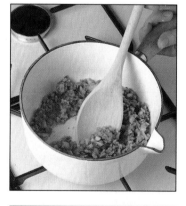

With floured hands, form mixture into 8 patties. Place them on baking sheet. Bake 15 to 20 minutes, until golden. Serve with lightly cooked vegetables.

Makes 4 servings.

Variation: Serve with a salad, if preferred.

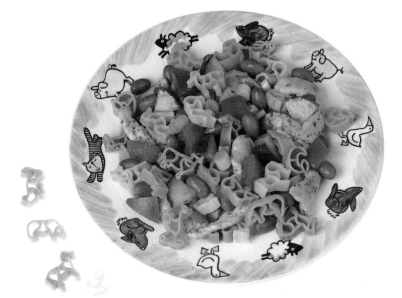

—CHICKEN & PASTA SALAD—

1/4 pound small pasta shapes, such as animals or shells
3/4 pound boneless chicken breasts
1 teaspoon Italian seasoning
2 tablespoons olive oil
3 tomatoes, seeded and diced
3 green onions, chopped
2-inch piece cucumber, diced
1 (7-oz.) can red kidney beans
4 teaspoons ketchup
2 teaspoons white-wine vinegar
Chopped fresh parsley, to garnish

Cook pasta in boiling salted water according to package directions. Drain well.

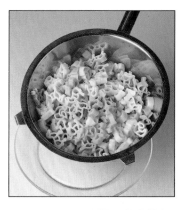

With a sharp knife, cut chicken into small strips. Sprinkle with Italian seasoning. In a nonstick skillet, heat half the oil. Add chicken and cook over medium heat 8 to 10 minutes, stirring occasionally, until cooked through. Transfer to a bowl.

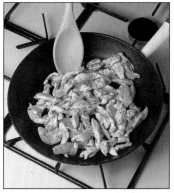

Stir in pasta, tomatoes, green onions and cucumber. Rinse and drain beans, then add to salad. Mix remaining oil with ketchup and vinegar. Add to salad and toss so all ingredients are well coated. Cover with plastic wrap and chill until required. Serve garnished with chopped fresh parsley.

Makes 4 servings.

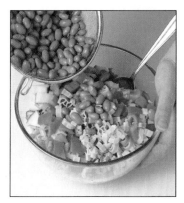

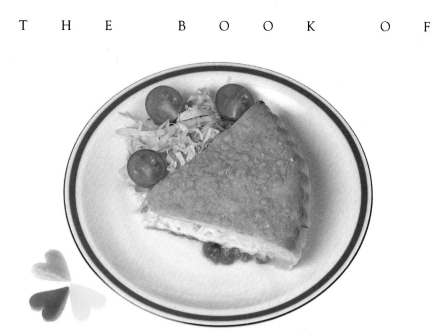

PIZZA PIE

1 (5-oz.) package pizza dough mix
4 tablespoons prepared pizza sauce
3/4 cup shredded mozzarella cheese (3 ounces)
3/4 cup shredded Cheddar cheese (3 ounces)
1 tablespoon butter or margarine
2 tablespoons freshly grated Parmesan cheese
Shredded lettuce and cherry tomato halves, to serve

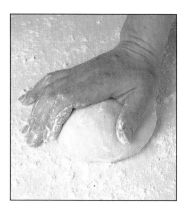

Grease a 7-inch quiche or tart pan. Prepare dough according to package directions. Turn out dough onto lightly floured surface and knead 5 minutes.

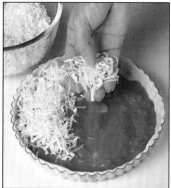

Shape two-thirds of the dough into a ball. Roll out thinly. Use to line quiche or tart pan. Spread pizza sauce over dough. Mix mozzarella and Cheddar cheeses together, then sprinkle over pizza sauce. Roll out remaining dough. Position dough over pie and pinch edges together to seal. Leave in a warm place 15 to 20 minutes, until dough has risen a little.

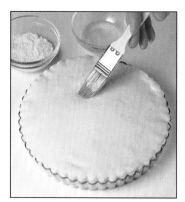

Meanwhile, preheat oven to 400F (205C). Melt butter, then brush over top of pie. Scatter Parmesan cheese on top. Bake about 20 minutes, until golden and crisp on top. Cut into wedges and serve with shredded lettuce and cherry tomatoes.

Makes 3 to 4 servings.

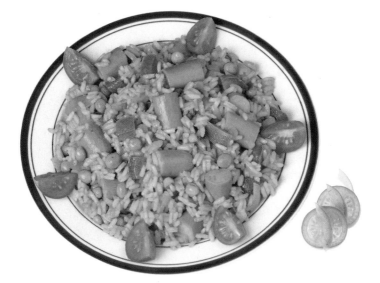

HOT DOG RISOTTO

2 tablespoons vegetable oil
1 large onion, chopped
1-1/2 cups long-grain rice
1 red or green bell pepper, chopped
2 cups hot chicken stock
1 (7-oz.) can tomatoes
8 hot dogs
3/4 cup frozen green peas
Salt and pepper
Tomato slices or wedges, to garnish

In a large saucepan, heat oil. Add onion and cook until softened, stirring occasionally. Stir in rice and bell pepper, and cook 1 minute, stirring constantly.

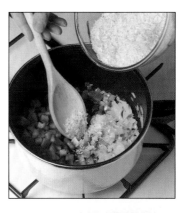

Pour in stock. Push tomatoes through a strainer into pan. Bring mixture to a boil, then reduce heat, cover and simmer 15 to 20 minutes, until the rice is tender and all liquid has been absorbed.

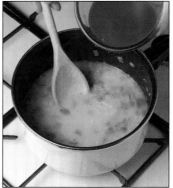

With a knife, cut hot dogs into 1/2-inch pieces. Add to risotto with peas, salt and pepper. Stir together over low heat 3 minutes longer. Serve hot, garnished with tomato slices or wedges.

Makes 4 servings.

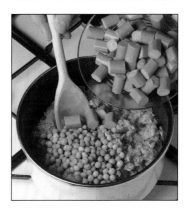

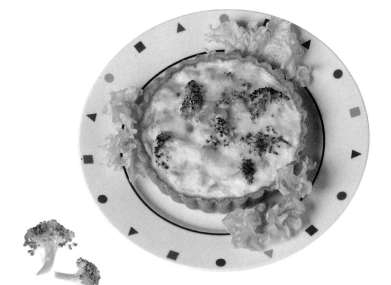

-TURKEY & BROCCOLI QUICHES-

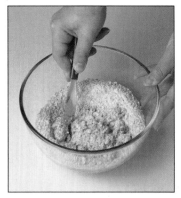

1-1/3 cups whole-wheat flour
Pinch of salt
1/3 cup butter or margarine, chilled
2 tablespoons vegetable oil
1/2 pound boneless turkey breast meat
6 ounces broccoli flowerets
1/2 cup shredded Gouda cheese (2 ounces)
3 eggs
1-1/4 cups milk
Salt and pepper
Lettuce leaves, to garnish

In a bowl, mix together flour and salt. Cut in butter until mixture resembles bread crumbs.

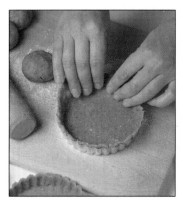

Add 1 tablespoon oil and 3 tablespoons water and mix to a dough. Divide dough into 6 pieces. Roll each piece out and use to line 6 (4-inch) quiche pans. Place on 2 baking sheets. Preheat oven to 375F (190C). With a knife, dice turkey meat. In nonstick pan, heat remaining oil. Add turkey and cook 4 to 5 minutes, until no longer pink. Set aside.

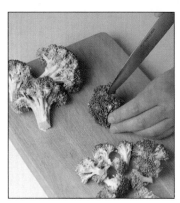

Trim broccoli into tiny flowerets. Blanch in boiling lightly salted water 2 minutes. Drain well. Divide cheese between pastry shells, then add turkey and broccoli. In a small bowl, beat eggs and milk together. Season with salt and pepper, then pour into quiches. Bake 25 to 30 minutes, until set. Remove from pans and serve warm or at room temperature. Garnish with lettuce leaves.

Makes 6 servings.

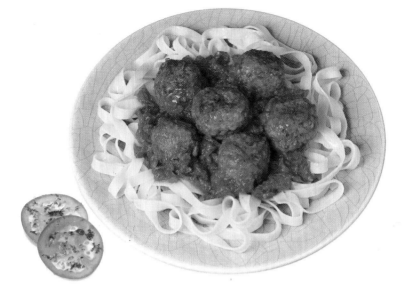

ITALIAN MEATBALLS

1 medium-thick slice whole-wheat bread
3 tablespoons milk
1 pound lean ground beef
1 garlic clove, crushed
1 tablespoon chopped fresh parsley
1 egg, beaten
Salt and pepper
1/4 cup all-purpose flour
2 tablespoons vegetable oil
1 (14-oz.) can tomatoes
1 teaspoon dried leaf oregano
1/2 teaspoon sugar

Remove crust from bread. Put bread into a small bowl, add milk and leave to soak.

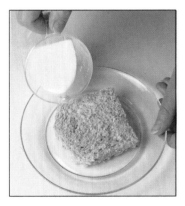

Into a bowl, put beef, garlic, parsley and egg. Add soaked bread, season with salt and pepper and mix until well blended. Divide into 20 small balls, rolling with wet hands. Dust each meatball with flour, shaking off any excess.

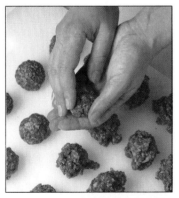

In a large skillet, heat oil. Add meatballs and fry until browned all over; cook in batches, if necessary. Lift out with a slotted spoon and transfer to a large saucepan. Crush tomatoes, then pour over meatballs. Add oregano and sugar, and simmer 20 to 25 minutes, until tomatoes and their juices have thickened to make a sauce. Serve with cooked pasta shapes or noodles.

Makes 4 servings.

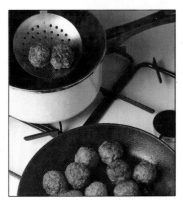

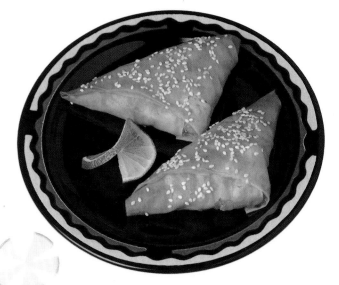

VEGETABLE SAMOSAS

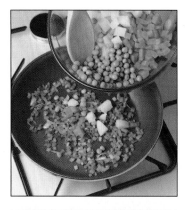

1 tablespoon vegetable oil
1 small onion, finely chopped
1 garlic clove, crushed
2 teaspoons mild curry powder
1-1/3 cups diced cooked potatoes
1/2 cup frozen green peas
1-1/3 cups diced cooked carrots
12 sheets filo pastry
1/4 cup butter or margarine, melted
Sesame seeds

In a medium-size saucepan, heat oil. Add onion and garlic and cook until softened. Stir in curry powder, and cook 1 minute. Mix in potatoes, peas and carrots. Let cool.

Preheat oven to 375F (190C). Grease 2 baking sheets. Brush a sheet of filo pastry with butter. Place 1 tablespoon filling in center of one end. Fold pastry over lengthwise. Brush with butter.

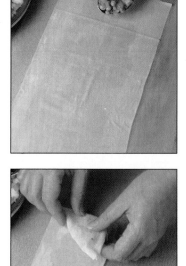

Take corner of rectangle and fold it over to make triangle. Fold stuffed portion away from you, keeping pastry's three-cornered shape. Continue folding, until you reach end of pastry. Fill and fold remaining pastry sheets the same way. Place on baking sheets, brush with butter and scatter sesame seeds over tops. Bake about 15 minutes, until golden and crisp. Serve hot.

Makes 12.

Note: Garnish with lime twists, if wished.

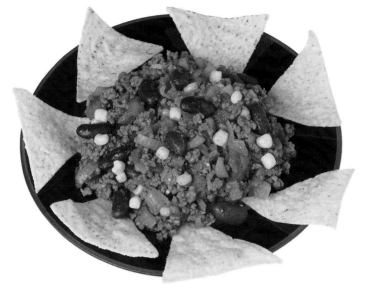

——————— MEXICAN SUPPER ———————

1 pound lean ground beef
1 onion, chopped
1 teaspoon mild chili powder
1 teaspoon ground cumin
1 (14-oz.) can chopped tomatoes
1 tablespoon tomato paste
1 (7-oz.) can red kidney beans, drained
1 cup frozen whole-kernel corn
Salt and pepper
Corn chips, to serve

Into a large, deep skillet, put beef, onion and spices. Cook 4 to 5 minutes, stirring, until meat is browned and onion is softened.

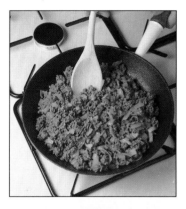

Stir in tomatoes and tomato paste, then cover and simmer 15 minutes.

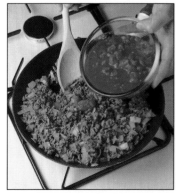

Stir in kidney beans and corn, and season with salt and pepper. Continue cooking 10 minutes longer, stirring occasionally. Serve with corn chips.

Makes 4 servings.

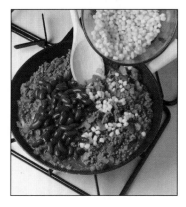

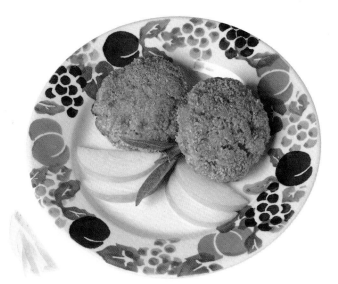

—SAUSAGE & APPLE BURGERS—

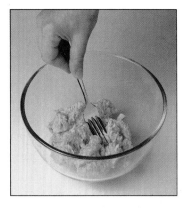

1 pound low-fat pork or turkey sausage meat
1/2 cup finely chopped onion
1 large cooking apple, grated
Pinch of Italian seasoning
Salt and pepper
2 tablespoons regular rolled oats
Apple slices and sage sprigs, to garnish

Preheat oven to 400F (205C). Grease a baking sheet. In a bowl, break up sausage meat with a fork.

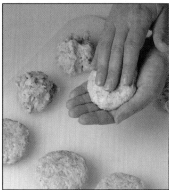

Add onion, apple, herbs, salt and pepper. Mix together until well blended. Shape into 8 balls and flatten slightly into patties.

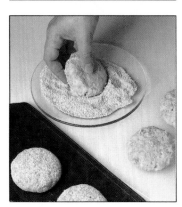

Coat each patty with oats, then place on baking sheet. Cook 25 to 30 minutes, until golden, turning them over halfway through cooking. Serve garnished with apple slices and sage sprigs.

Makes 4 servings.

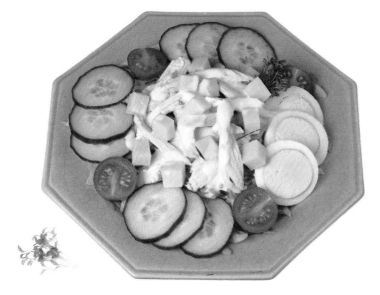

——— CHEF'S SALAD ———

1/2 small head iceberg lettuce, shredded
2 carrots, grated
2 eggs, hard-cooked
1/2 cucumber, sliced
8 cherry tomatoes, halved
1 cup shredded cooked chicken
3/4 cup diced Edam or Gouda cheese
Radish or mustard sprouts
DRESSING:
1/4 cup plain yogurt
1/4 cup mayonnaise
2 teaspoons lemon juice
1 tablespoon orange juice

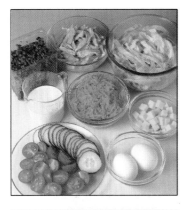

Put lettuce into 1 large serving bowl or 4 individual salad bowls. Top with grated carrots. Slice eggs and arrange around side of the bowl (or bowls) with cucumber and tomatoes. Put shredded chicken in middle and top with cheese.

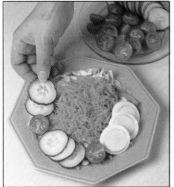

To make dressing, in a small bowl, mix all ingredients together until well blended. Drizzle dressing over the salad, then garnish with sprouts.

Makes 4 servings.

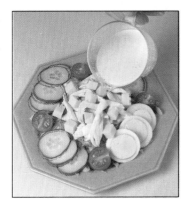

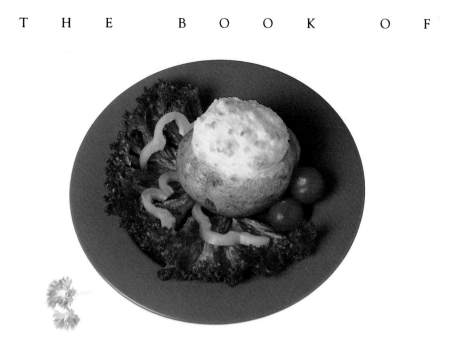

—— TWICE-BAKED POTATOES ——

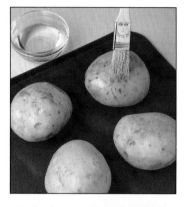

4 baking potatoes
Vegetable oil for brushing
2 tablespoons butter or margarine
3 eggs, separated
3/4 cup shredded Cheddar cheese
Salt and pepper
Cherry tomatoes, lettuce leaves and bell pepper strips,
   to serve

Preheat oven to 400F (205C). With a fork, prick potatoes all over. Brush skins lightly with oil. Bake 45 to 60 minutes, until softened.

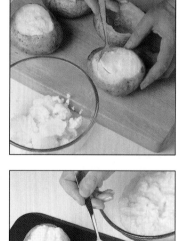

With a knife, cut off tops of potatoes. Scoop out cooked centers and put into a bowl, making sure skins are not pierced. Mash potatoes with butter, then beat in egg yolks, cheese, salt and pepper.

Beat egg whites until stiff but not dry, then fold into mashed potatoes. Spoon back into potato skins. Bake 10 to 15 minutes longer, until puffed and golden on top. Serve with cherry tomatoes, lettuce leaves and bell pepper strips.

Makes 4 servings.

Variations: Stir in 1/4 cup chopped cooked ham, or 1 tablespoon chopped sweet pickle, if desired.

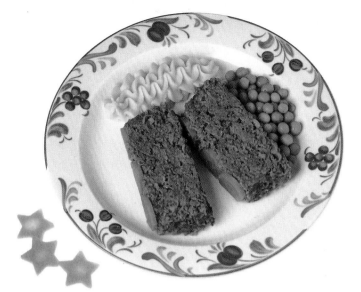

─── TASTY MEAT LOAF ───

6 ounces carrots
1 pound lean ground beef
1 cup fresh white or whole-wheat bread crumbs
1/3 cup finely chopped onion
1/2 teaspoon prepared mustard
2 tablespoons tomato paste
1 teaspoon Italian seasoning
1 egg, beaten
Salt and pepper
Green peas and buttered noodles, to serve

Preheat oven to 350F (175C). Grease and line an 8" x 4" loaf pan with waxed paper. With a knife, thinly slice enough carrots to line bottom of pan.

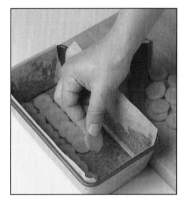

Into a bowl, grate remaining carrots. Add remaining ingredients. Mix well.

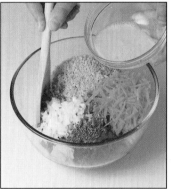

Spoon mixture into pan and level the surface with a spatula. Cover top with foil. Bake 1 hour, until firm. To serve, turn out meat loaf onto a flat plate, then peel off lining paper. Serve hot or at room temperature. Serve with peas and noodles.

Makes 4 to 5 servings.

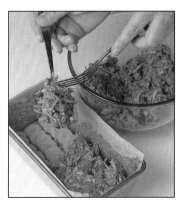

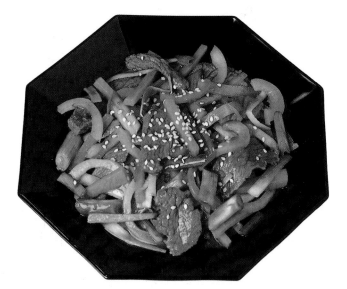

— DANIEL'S FAVORITE STIR-FRY —

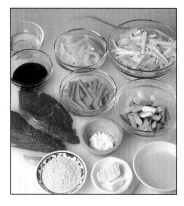

3/4 pound beef sirloin steak
2 tablespoons soy sauce
1 tablespoon creamed coconut
5 tablespoons boiling water
2 tablespoons vegetable oil
1 garlic clove, crushed
1 large carrot, cut into matchsticks
1 leek, shredded
1 red or yellow bell pepper, thinly sliced
5 green onions, chopped
2 teaspoons cornstarch
3 tablespoons orange juice
Sesame seeds
Cooked rice or noodles

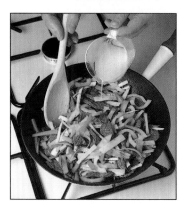

With a sharp knife, cut steak into thin strips. Put into a bowl with 1 tablespoon of the soy sauce and mix together. Dissolve creamed coconut in boiling water, then set aside. In a large skillet or wok, heat oil. Add steak and garlic and stir-fry 3 to 4 minutes, until steak is almost brown all over.

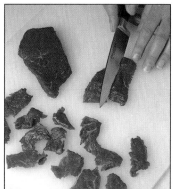

Add carrot, leek and bell pepper and stir-fry 3 minutes longer. Add coconut mixture, remaining soy sauce and green onions, then bring to a simmer, stirring constantly. Blend cornstarch with orange juice. Add to skillet and cook to thicken sauce, stirring constantly. Sprinkle over the sesame seeds. Serve hot with rice or noodles.

Makes 4 servings.

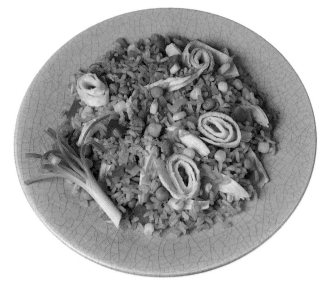

CHICKEN FRIED RICE

1-1/2 cups long-grain brown rice
3 tablespoons vegetable oil
1 egg
1 tablespoon water
1 small onion, finely chopped
1 red bell pepper, chopped
1-1/2 cups shredded cooked chicken (8 ounces)
1/3 cup frozen green peas, thawed
1/3 cup frozen whole-kernel corn, thawed
1 tablespoon soy sauce
Green onions, to garnish

Cook rice in boiling water according to package directions until tender; drain, if necessary.

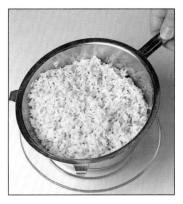

In a medium-size skillet, heat 2 tablespoons of the oil. Beat egg with water, then add to skillet and cook until set. Turn out omelet onto a board, then roll up and cut into thin strips; set aside. In a large skillet, heat remaining oil. Add onion and bell pepper, and cook 2 to 3 minutes.

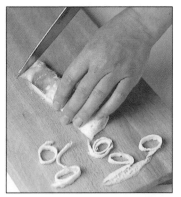

Stir in rice and stir-fry over low heat 3 to 4 minutes. Add chicken, peas, corn and soy sauce and continue stir-frying 3 minutes longer. Add omelet strips to fried rice and toss together before serving. Garnish with green onions.

Makes 4 servings.

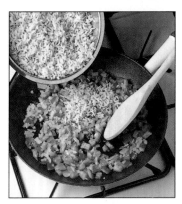

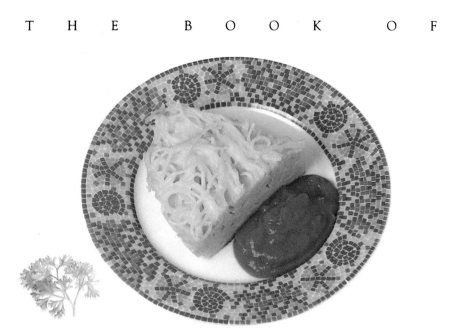

SPAGHETTI FRITTATA

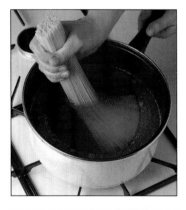

1/2 pound spaghetti
2 tablespoons olive oil
Salt
1 onion, finely chopped
4 eggs
1 cup shredded Cheddar cheese (4 ounces)
1/2 garlic clove, crushed
2 teaspoons all-purpose flour
1-1/4 cups canned tomatoes, sieved with some of the
 liquid drained off

Cook spaghetti in boiling salted water according to package directions until just tender to the bite. Drain.

In a medium-size skillet, heat 2 teaspoons of the oil. Add half the onion and cook 2 to 3 minutes, until softened. Remove skillet from heat; set aside. In a large bowl, beat eggs, then stir in cheese and cooked onion. Season with a little salt, then mix in spaghetti. Turn mixture into skillet and place over medium-low heat. Cook about 10 minutes, until set.

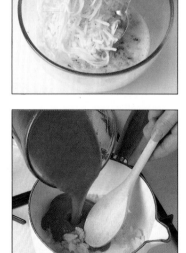

Meanwhile, preheat broiler. In a small saucepan, heat remaining oil. Add remaining uncooked onion and garlic and cook 2 to 3 minutes, until softened. Stir in flour and chopped tomatoes, then bring to a simmer, stirring constantly. Cook sauce 4 to 5 minutes longer. Once frittata is set, place under medium-hot broiler until lightly browned. Cut into wedges and serve with the sauce.

Makes 4 servings.

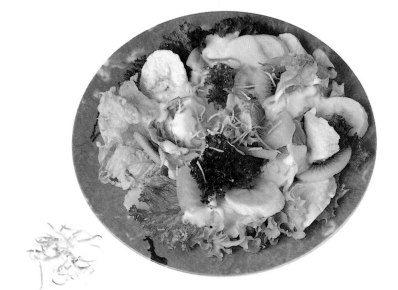

—COCONUT CHICKEN SALAD—

Lettuce leaves
2 cooked chicken breasts
2 large bananas
1 kiwifruit, peeled and sliced
2 canned pineapple slices, drained and cut into pieces
DRESSING:
2/3 cup shredded coconut
3/4 cup boiling water
2 tablespoons mayonnaise
Pineapple juice (optional)
Toasted coconut, to garnish

First, make the dressing. Into a saucepan, put coconut with water. Simmer 2 minutes.

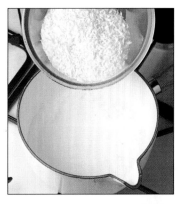

Pour coconut mixture into a food processor or blender and process until finely chopped. Press the pulp through a strainer, pressing with back of spoon to extract all liquid. Reserve coconut pulp.

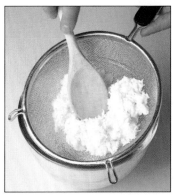

Wash and dry lettuce leaves, then arrange on 4 serving plates. Discard skin and bones from chicken, then cut meat into small pieces. Thickly slice bananas. Arrange over lettuce along with chicken, kiwifruit and pineapple. Beat mayonnaise into coconut milk, adding a little reserved coconut for a thicker dressing, or a little pineapple juice for a thinner dressing. Spoon over salad. Garnish with toasted coconut.

Makes 4 servings.

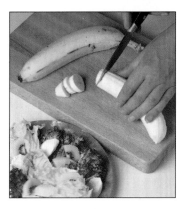

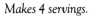

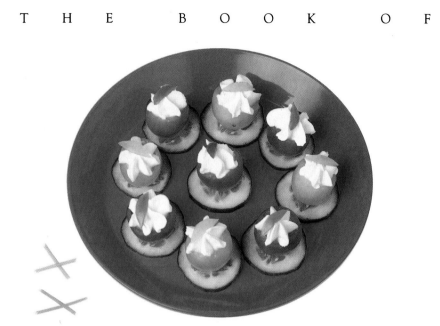

——— TOMATO FLOWERS ———

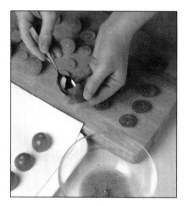

1/2 pound cherry tomatoes, red or yellow, if available
3/4 cup low-fat cream cheese (6 ounces)
1/2 cucumber, sliced
Fresh chives, to garnish

With a sharp knife, cut off tomato tops and reserve. Scoop out tomato centers, then place upside down on a double thickness of paper towels to drain.

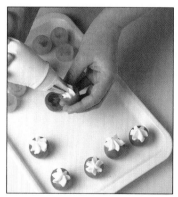

In a small bowl, beat cheese to soften. Place in a pastry bag fitted with a small star tip. Pipe cheese into tomatoes.

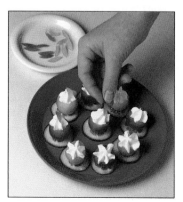

Arrange cucumber slices on a serving plate. Place tomatoes on top. Cut tiny pieces of tomato from reserved tops and use to decorate stuffed tomatoes. Garnish with chives.

Makes 6 to 8 servings.

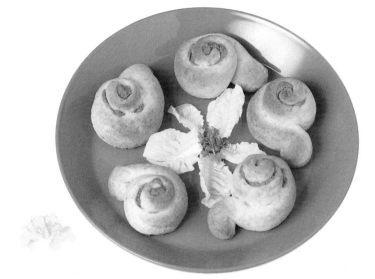

PEANUT SNAILS

1-1/2 cups self-rising flour
1/2 teaspoon mustard powder
1/3 cup margarine
1/2 cup shredded Cheddar cheese (2 ounces)
3 tablespoons milk
Peanut butter
Lettuce leaves and radish or mustard sprouts, to serve

Preheat oven to 375F (190C). Grease a baking sheet. Into a bowl, sift flour and mustard powder. Cut in margarine until mixture resembles fine bread crumbs. Stir in cheese, then milk to make a fairly soft dough.

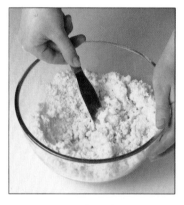

Turn out dough onto a floured surface and knead lightly until smooth. Roll dough into a rope shape about 12 inches long. Cut into 20 equal slices. Roll out each slice into a thin rope shape about 6 inches long. Gently press three-quarters of the length to make dough about 1/2 inch wide.

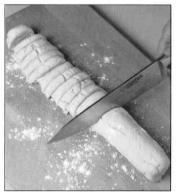

Spread a little peanut butter along flattened surface, then roll up toward unflattened end to make a snail shape. Form a head at the end. Transfer to baking sheet. Repeat with remaining dough. Bake 12 to 15 minutes, until golden. Cool on a wire rack. Serve with lettuce leaves and sprouts.

Makes 20.

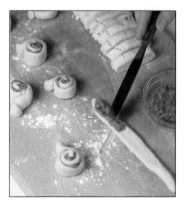

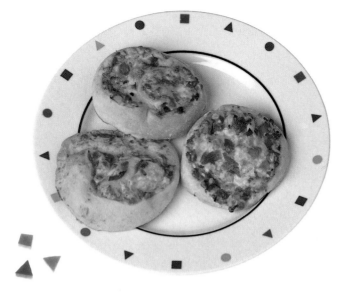

PIZZA SWIRLS

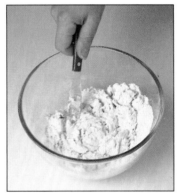

2 cups bread flour
Pinch of salt
1 (1/4-oz.) package active dry yeast
2/3 cup canned chopped tomatoes, drained
2 tablespoons tomato paste
1 garlic clove, crushed
1 teaspoon dried leaf oregano
1 (7-oz.) can tuna, drained and flaked
1 red or green bell pepper, finely chopped
1 small onion, finely chopped
3/4 cup shredded mozzarella cheese (3 ounces)

Into a bowl, sift flour and salt. Add yeast and 3/4 cup plus 2 tablespoons warm water (130F, 55C). Mix to a soft dough.

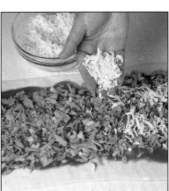

Turn out dough onto a lightly floured surface. Knead 10 minutes, until smooth. Roll out to a 16″ x 8″ rectangle. Mix tomatoes, tomato paste, garlic and oregano together. Spread over dough. Mix tuna with bell pepper and onion, then spoon over the tomato mixture. Sprinkle with cheese.

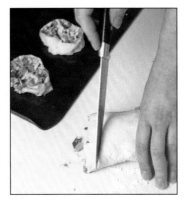

Grease a baking sheet. Roll up dough from a long side, then cut into 1/2-inch slices. Place slices, cut sides up, on baking sheets and leave in a warm place 15 minutes. Meanwhile, preheat oven to 375F (190C). Bake pizza swirls 15 minutes, until golden-brown. Serve warm.

Makes 25 to 30.

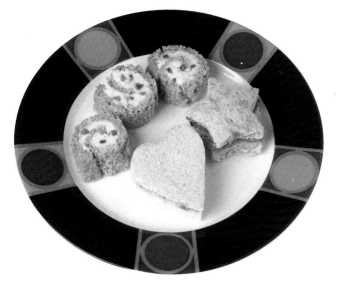

PARTY SANDWICHES

PINWHEELS:
4 slices whole-wheat bread
1/2 cup cream cheese (4 ounces), softened
3/4 cup shredded Cheddar cheese (3 ounces)
2 tablespoons finely chopped red bell pepper
HEARTS:
6 slices white or whole-wheat bread
1 (3-1/2-oz.) can tuna, drained
2 tablespoons low-fat cream cheese, softened
STARS:
6 slices mixed-grain bread
12 small slices salami or ham
Cucumber slices

Margarine or butter, softened, for spreading

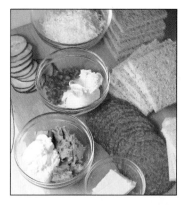

To make pinwheel sandwiches, with a knife, remove crusts from bread and roll slices with a rolling pin to flatten slightly. Spread bread with a little margarine. Make filling by mixing cheeses and bell pepper together. Spread filling over bread, then roll up each slice like a jellyroll. To make heart-shaped sandwiches, cut out heart shapes from the bread slices, then spread a little margarine on one side. Mix tuna and cream cheese together until combined. Use to fill heart shapes.

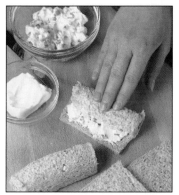

To make star-shaped sandwiches, cut out stars from bread, salami and cucumber. Lightly spread bread with margarine, then make up each star with a piece of salami and cucumber. Cover with plastic wrap and refrigerate all sandwiches until needed. To serve pinwheels, unwrap and cut each into 4 slices. Serve with stars and hearts.

Makes 40 assorted sandwiches.

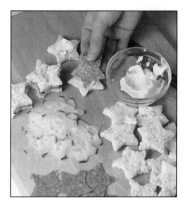

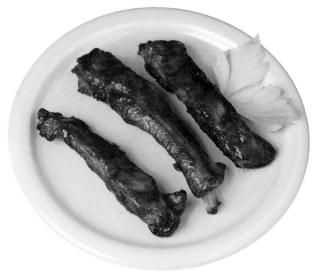

STICKY RIBS

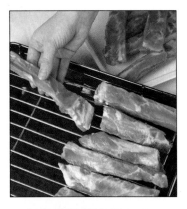

1-1/2 pounds pork spareribs
5 tablespoons ketchup
2 tablespoons honey
1 tablespoon soy sauce
1 tablespoon wine vinegar
1 tablespoon Worcestershire sauce
2 tablespoons orange juice
Celery leaves, to garnish

Preheat oven to 400F (205C). Cut ribs into single rib pieces. Arrange on a roasting rack set in a roasting pan. Pour a little water into pan. Bake ribs 25 minutes.

Meanwhile, in a bowl, mix remaining ingredients together. Brush the ribs on both sides with glaze. Reduce oven temperature to 350F (175C), then continue cooking ribs 15 minutes longer.

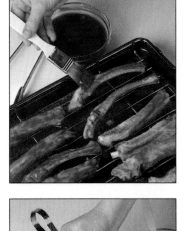

Turn ribs over, brush again with glaze and cook 15 to 20 minutes longer, until golden-brown. Garnish with celery leaves. Serve hot with a salad.

Makes 6 servings.

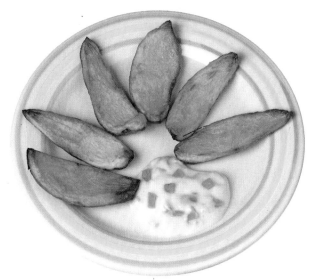

———— PARTY POTATO SKINS ————

2-1/4 pounds red potatoes
3 tablespoons olive oil
Salt
CHEESE & HAM SAUCE:
1 tablespoon butter
1 tablespoon all-purpose flour
1-1/4 cups milk
1/2 cup shredded Cheddar cheese (2 ounces)
1/3 cup minced cooked ham
Pinch of red (cayenne) pepper (optional)

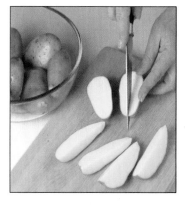

With a knife, cut unpeeled potatoes lengthwise into even wedges. Cook in boiling water 5 minutes, then drain.

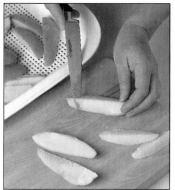

Preheat oven to 425F (220C). Cool potato wedges until cool enough to handle, then cut out the centers, leaving about 1/2-inch shells. Place skins on a baking sheet and brush with oil, then sprinkle with salt. Bake about 20 minutes, until crisp.

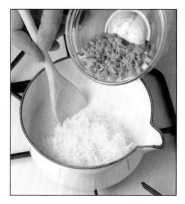

Meanwhile, make sauce. In a small saucepan, melt butter. Stir in flour, then gradually stir in milk. Cook, stirring constantly, until thickened. Stir in cheese and ham. Stir until cheese melts, and season with cayenne, if desired. Serve warm with potato skins.

Makes 6 to 8 servings.

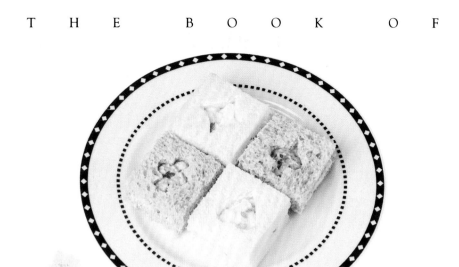

—PLAYING CARD SANDWICHES—

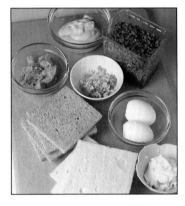

4 slices whole-wheat bread, crusts removed
4 slices white bread, crusts removed
Margarine or butter, softened
SALMON FILLING:
1 tablespoon mayonnaise
2 teaspoons lemon juice
1 (3-1/2-oz.) can red salmon, drained, skin and bones
    removed
1/2 carton radish or mustard sprouts, trimmed
EGG FILLING:
2 eggs, hard-cooked
1 tablespoon mayonnaise
2 green onions, finely chopped

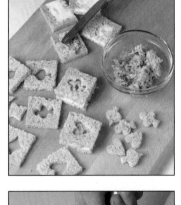

With a knife, cut each slice of bread into quarters. Cut out playing card symbols from centers of half of the quarters. To make Salmon Filling, in a small bowl, beat mayonnaise and lemon juice together. Stir in salmon until combined, then stir in sprouts. Lightly spread margarine over whole squares of whole-wheat bread. Spread Salmon Filling on top, then cover with cut-out whole-wheat quarters.

To make Egg Filling, in a small bowl, mash eggs into small pieces with a fork. Stir in mayonnaise and onions. Make up egg sandwiches like salmon sandwiches, using the white bread.

Makes 16 sandwiches.

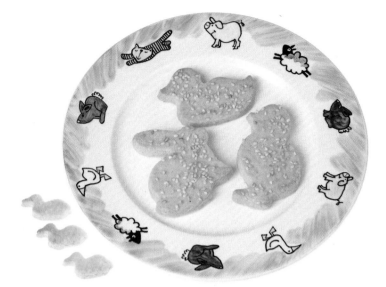

—ANIMAL CHEESE CRACKERS—

1 cup all-purpose flour
1/2 teaspoon mustard powder
1/4 cup butter, chilled
1/2 cup shredded sharp Cheddar cheese (2 ounces)
1 egg, beaten
Sesame seeds

Preheat oven to 350F (175C). Grease 2 baking sheets. Into a bowl, sift flour and mustard. Cut in butter until mixture resembles bread crumbs.

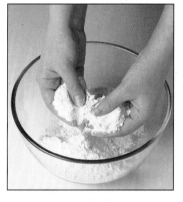

Stir in cheese, then add 2 tablespoons of the beaten egg and mix together to make a smooth dough. Turn dough out onto a floured surface and knead lightly. Roll out to about 1 inch thick.

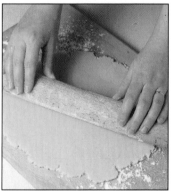

Using animal-shaped cookie cutters, cut out crackers, rerolling trimmings. Place on baking sheets. Brush tops with remaining beaten egg and sprinkle with sesame seeds. Bake 12 to 15 minutes, until golden. Cool on a wire rack.

Makes about 18.

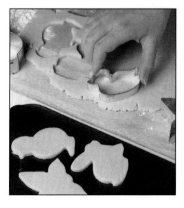

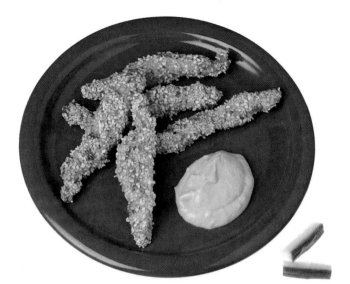

— SESAME CHICKEN FINGERS —

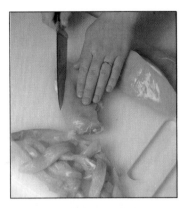

1-1/2 pounds skinless, boneless chicken breasts
3 tablespoons all-purpose flour
2 teaspoons curry powder and paprika, mixed
Salt and pepper
2 eggs
1-1/2 cups sesame seeds
SAUCE:
1/4 cup mayonnaise
2 teaspoons tomato paste
2 tomatoes, peeled, seeded and chopped
1 small garlic clove, crushed

Preheat oven to 400F (205C). Grease a baking sheet. With a knife, cut chicken into strips about 1/2 inch wide.

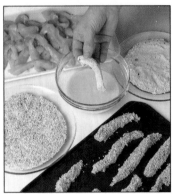

In a bowl, mix flour and curry powder and paprika together. Season with salt and pepper. Beat eggs and pour into a shallow dish. Dust chicken strips with spicy flour mixture, then dip into eggs. Toss strips in sesame seeds, then transfer to baking sheet. Bake 20 to 25 minutes.

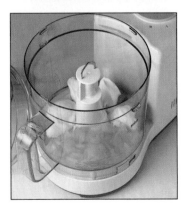

Meanwhile, put all sauce ingredients into a food processor or blender and process until smooth. Serve with cooked chicken strips.

Makes 6 to 8 servings.

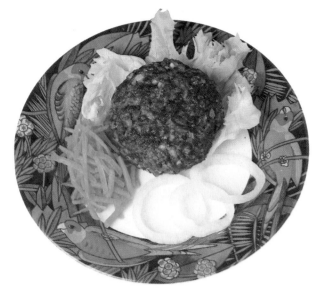

——— SURPRISE HAMBURGERS ———

1-1/4 pounds lean ground beef
1 small onion, finely chopped
1 teaspoon Italian seasoning
2/3 cup rolled oats
1 egg, beaten
Salt and pepper
1 (3-oz.) piece cheese, such as Gouda
1 tablespoon vegetable oil
Grated carrots, lettuce leaves and onion rings, to serve

Into a bowl, put beef, onion, herbs and oats. Mix together to break up beef. Add egg, salt and pepper; stir until combined.

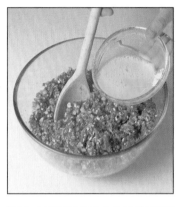

With floured hands, divide mixture into 6 balls, then flatten each on a board or flat surface. With a knife, cut cheese into 6 pieces. Place a piece in middle of each meat patty. Preheat broiler.

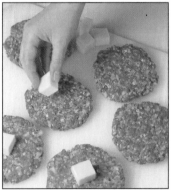

Carefully enclose each cheese piece in meat mixture, then form into patties. Brush with oil, place under a medium-hot broiler and broil 4 to 5 minutes on each side, until browned. Serve with carrots, lettuce leaves and onion rings.

Makes 6 servings.

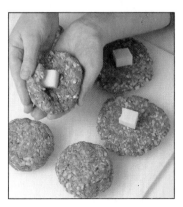

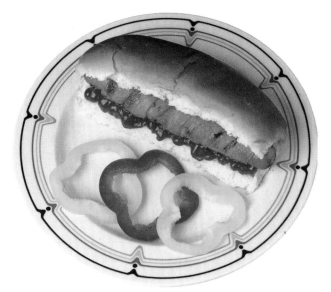

HOT DOG TWISTS

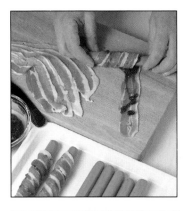

8 bacon slices
2 to 3 tablespoons barbecue sauce
8 hot dogs
8 hot dog buns
Ketchup or extra barbecue sauce, to serve
Bell pepper rings, to garnish

Spread each bacon slice with sauce. Wrap around each hot dog. Preheat broiler.

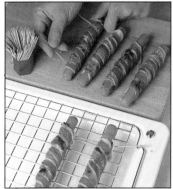

Secure each end of the bacon with a wooden pick. Arrange on a broiler pan and place as far away from heat as possible.

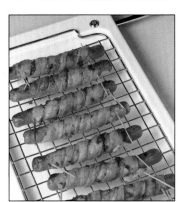

Cook hot dog twists until bacon is crisp and just lightly browned, turning frequently during cooking. Remove wooden picks. Serve in split, hot dog buns with extra ketchup or barbecue sauce. Garnish with bell pepper rings.

Makes 8 servings.

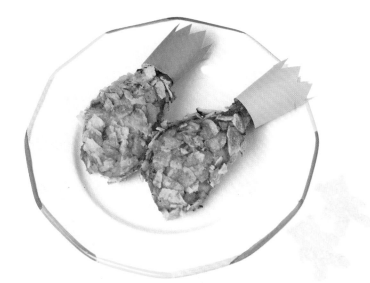

—SPICY CHICKEN DRUMSTICKS—

8 chicken legs
2 tablespoons ketchup
1 tablespoon honey
1 tablespoon mild chili powder
2 (1-oz.) bags potato chips

Preheat oven to 375F (190C). With a sharp knife, remove skin from each leg.

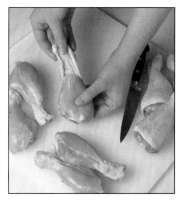

In a small bowl, mix ketchup, honey and chili powder together. Brush over legs.

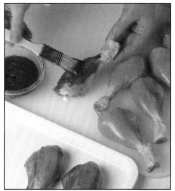

Lightly crush potato chips and put in a shallow dish. Roll legs in potato chips to coat. Place coated legs on a rack set in a roasting pan. Bake 30 minutes, until golden. Pierce each drumstick with a skewer to check that the juices run clear; if still pink, bake a little longer, before testing again.

Makes 8.

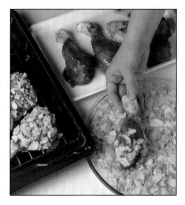

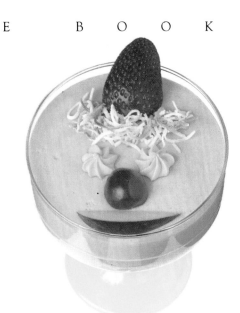

——— CLOWN TRIFLES ———

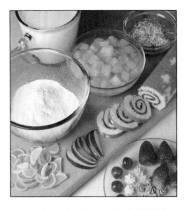

6 slices from a jellyroll
1 (14-oz.) can fruit cocktail
1 package instant pudding and pie mix (butterscotch,
    peach or strawberry flavor)
Milk
TO DECORATE:
6 tablespoons shredded coconut, lightly toasted
6 large strawberries
12 candy stars
6 candied cherries
6 red apple slices
Candy orange and lemon slices

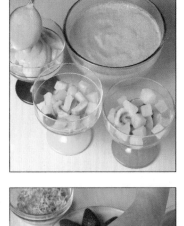

Place a jellyroll slice in bottom of 6 small dishes or cups. Drain fruit cocktail, then spoon over jellyroll slices. Make up pudding with milk as directed on package. Spoon pudding evenly over fruit.

When pudding is set, decorate each trifle to look like a clown. Arrange coconut to look like hair, a strawberry for a hat, candy stars for eyes, a candied cherry for the nose and an apple slice for the mouth. Place on a plate and arrange orange and lemon slices around each dish to look like a ruffled collar.

Makes 6 servings.

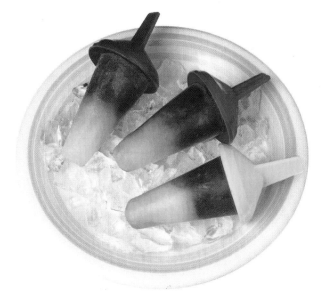

─────── RAINBOW POPS ───────

1/2 cup orange juice
3 ounces fresh raspberries or strawberries
1 teaspoon sugar
1/4 cup grape juice

Into a plastic mold or individual molds, pour orange juice. Place in freezer and leave until frozen.

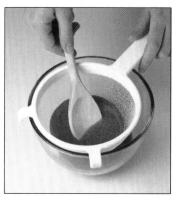

Put raspberries or strawberries, sugar and 1/4 cup cold water into a food processor or blender and process until smooth. Pour through a strainer, then pour over frozen orange juice. Return to freezer about 1 hour, until almost frozen.

Mix grape juice with 1/4 cup cold water, then pour over strawberry or raspberry layer. Insert the holders and put back into freezer until solid. To unmold, dip each mold in a bowl of hot water for a few seconds, then pull off. Serve at once.

Makes about 4, depending on size of molds.

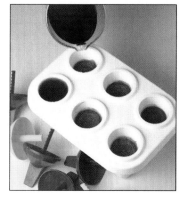

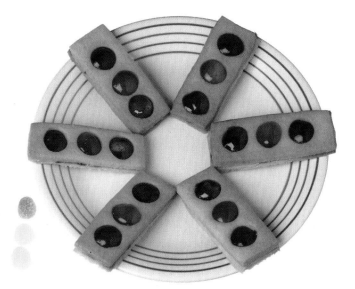

— TRAFFIC LIGHT COOKIES —

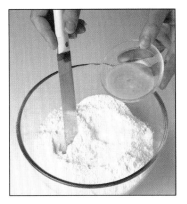

2 cups all-purpose flour
1/2 cup powdered sugar
2/3 cup butter, chilled
1 egg yolk
4 tablespoons strawberry jam
2 tablespoons apricot jam
2 tablespoons lime marmalade

Into a bowl, sift flour and powdered sugar. Cut in butter until mixture resembles bread crumbs. Add egg yolk and mix to form a dough. Turn out dough onto a floured surface and knead until smooth. Cover with plastic wrap and refrigerate at least 30 minutes.

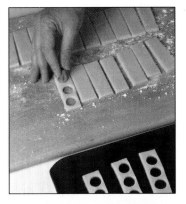

Preheat oven to 325F (165C). Grease a baking sheet. Cut dough in half. Roll out one half to a 10″ x 6″ rectangle. Cut in half lengthwise, then cut each half crosswise into 10 (1-inch) strips. Place on baking sheet. Repeat with remaining dough, cutting into strips as before. Cut out 3 circles from each strip; discard dough circles. Transfer strips to baking sheet. Bake in oven 12 minutes, until lightly golden. Cool on baking sheet.

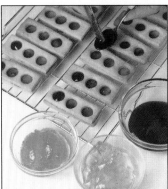

Using half the strawberry jam, spread a thin layer over plain cookies. Place cookies with holes on top. Strain remaining strawberry jam and fill top hole of each cookie. Repeat with apricot jam and lime marmalade in remaining holes to represent traffic lights.

Makes 20.

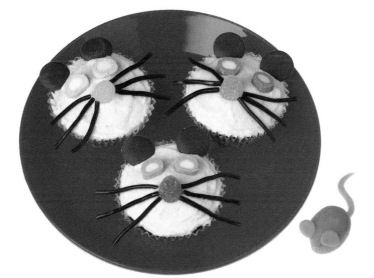

MERRY MICE CAKES

1 cup self-rising flour
1/4 cup unsweetened cocoa powder
1/2 cup margarine, softened
3/4 cup packed light brown sugar
2 eggs, beaten
2 tablespoons milk
DECORATIONS:
1 cup powdered sugar, sifted
6 tablespoons butter, softened
Chocolate buttons
Gumdrops
Licorice strands and candies

Preheat oven to 350F (175C). Into a bowl, put all cake ingredients. Beat until smooth.

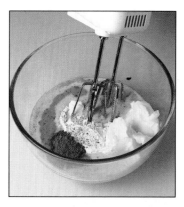

Divide cake batter evenly among 20 paper cupcake cups placed in 2 (12-cup) muffin pans; place water in unused cups. Bake about 15 minutes, until firm to the touch. Cool on a wire rack. Trim tops to flatten if there are peaks.

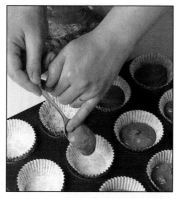

To decorate, in a small bowl, beat powdered sugar and butter together until light and fluffy. Spread over tops of cakes. Attach 2 chocolate buttons on each cake for ears, and place a gumdrop for a nose. Cut slices of licorice candies to make eyes. Cut pieces of licorice strands to make whiskers and insert 3 on each side of candy nose.

Makes 20.

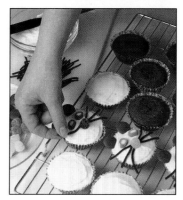

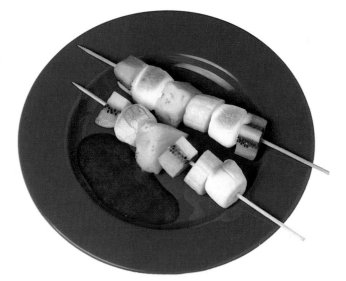

MARSHMALLOW-FRUIT KABOBS

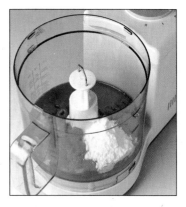

2 firm bananas
2 thick slices fresh pineapple
2 kiwifruit, cut into 3/4-inch pieces
24 marshmallows
1 tablespoon honey
1 tablespoon lemon juice
RASPBERRY SAUCE:
1/2 pound raspberries, fresh or frozen, thawed if frozen
Juice of 1 orange
1 tablespoon powdered sugar

In a food processor or blender, process raspberries, orange juice and powdered sugar
until smooth. Press through a strainer.

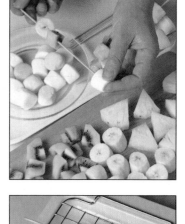

Preheat broiler. With a knife, cut bananas
into thick slices and pineapple into chunks.
Thread all fruit onto 12 oiled bamboo
skewers, alternating with marshmallows.
In a small bowl, combine honey and lemon
juice, then brush all over fruit.

Cook kabobs under medium-hot broiler until
marshmallows begin to color, turning once
during broiling. Serve with raspberry sauce.

Makes 12.

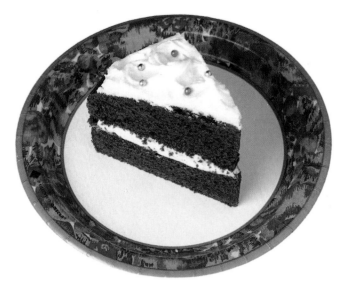

DEVIL'S FOOD CAKE

2 cups self-rising flour
1/2 cup unsweetened cocoa powder
2/3 cup butter, softened
1-1/2 cups packed dark brown sugar
3 eggs, beaten
2/3 cup milk
1 teaspoon vanilla extract
FROSTING:
1 egg white
3/4 cup sugar
1/4 teaspoon cream of tartar
1/2 teaspoon vanilla extract

Preheat oven to 350F (175C). Grease and line an 8-inch springform pan. Into medium-size bowl, sift flour and cocoa powder.

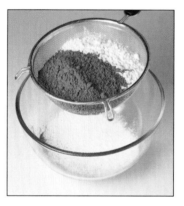

In another bowl, cream butter and sugar together until soft and fluffy. Beat in eggs, a little at a time. Stir in flour mixture until smooth, then beat in milk and vanilla. Spoon batter into pan and smooth top with a metal spatula. Bake about 40 minutes, until a wooden pick inserted in center comes out clean. Cool 10 minutes in pan, then turn out cake, peel off lining paper and transfer to a wire rack to cool completely.

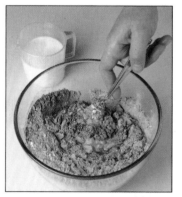

In a small heatproof bowl over a pan of simmering water, combine all frosting ingredients with 2 tablespoons cold water. Beat about 10 minutes, until smooth, white and standing in peaks. With a serrated knife, cut cake in half horizontally and level top, if needed. Sandwich together with half of the frosting; frost top and side with remaining frosting. Let stand about 1 hour to harden.

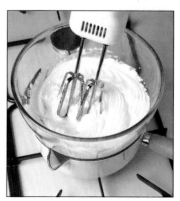

Makes 8 to 10 servings.

Variation: Decorate with candies, if desired.

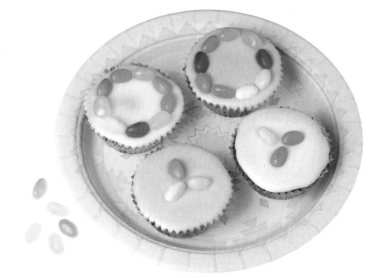

CUPCAKES

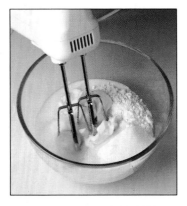

1 cup self-rising flour
1/2 cup sugar
1/2 cup margarine, softened
2 eggs
2 tablespoons milk
1 teaspoon vanilla extract
FROSTING:
1-1/2 cups powdered sugar
3 or 4 teaspoons water
Few drops of food coloring (optional)
Jellybeans or other candies, to decorate

Preheat oven to 350F (175C). In a medium-size bowl, beat together all cake ingredients until blended.

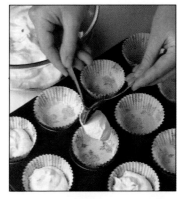

Using 2 spoons, divide batter among 20 paper cupcake cups placed in 2 (12-cup) muffin pans; put water in unused cups. Bake 15 minutes, until golden. Transfer to a wire rack to cool.

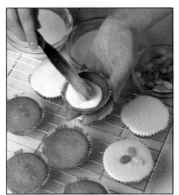

To make frosting, into a bowl, sift powdered sugar, then mix in just enough water to give a smooth consistency for coating. Tint some frosting with a small amount of coloring, if desired. Frost cupcakes and decorate as desired, while frosting is still soft. Let set before serving.

Makes 20.

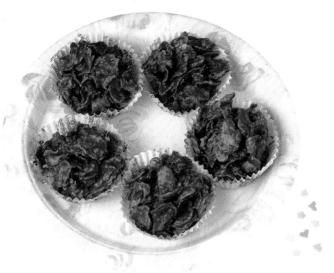

CRISPY CRACKLES

1/4 cup margarine or butter
2 tablespoons light corn syrup
4 ounces milk chocolate
3 cups cornflakes

In a medium-size saucepan, combine margarine or butter, corn syrup and chocolate. Place over low heat, stirring, until chocolate melts.

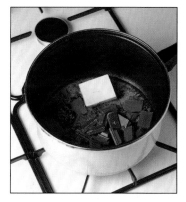

Remove pan from heat, then stir in cornflakes, stirring until cornflakes are evenly coated.

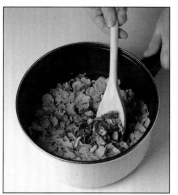

Put 12 paper cupcake cups into a muffin pan. Spoon in cornflake mixture. Refrigerate until set.

Makes 12.

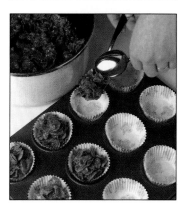

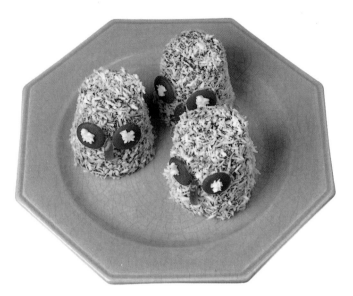

OWL MADELEINES

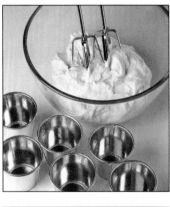

1/2 cup margarine, softened
1/2 cup sugar
1 cup self-rising flour
2 eggs, beaten
1/2 teaspoon vanilla extract
2/3 cup shredded coconut
1/4 cup strawberry or raspberry jam
2 tablespoons butter, softened
1/3 cup powdered sugar
16 chocolate buttons or drops
2 candied cherries

Grease 8 dariole molds, muffin cups or ramekins. Into a medium-size bowl, put margarine, sugar, flour, eggs and vanilla. Beat until smooth.

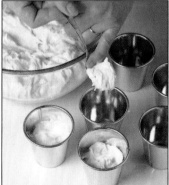

Preheat oven to 350F (175C). Spoon cake batter into molds or cups, filling each one half full. If using dariole molds or ramekins, place on a baking sheet after filling. Bake 15 to 18 minutes, until cakes feel firm when pressed. Remove from oven, run a round-bladed knife around inside of cups, then turn out cakes and transfer to a wire rack to cool. Trim so all cakes are the same height.

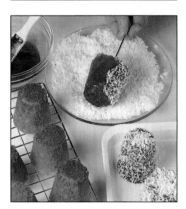

In a small plate, spread out coconut. In a small saucepan, melt jam with 1 tablespoon water. Push a skewer into each cake. Brush with melted jam, then roll in coconut until well coated. Put cakes, narrow ends up, on a plate. Beat butter and powdered sugar together. Use this mixture to attach 2 chocolate buttons to each cake for eyes. Pipe a spot of frosting in center of each eye. Complete owls with cherry pieces for beaks.

Makes 8.

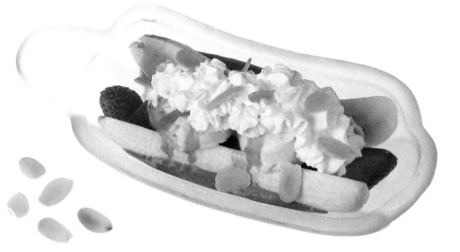

BANANA SPLITS

2 ounces chocolate candy bars, broken in pieces
6 tablespoons half and half
4 ripe bananas
a little lemon juice
8 scoops vanilla or chocolate ice cream
8 large strawberries, sliced
Whipped cream in aerosol can
1 tablespoon sliced almonds, lightly toasted

To make sauce, in a small heatproof bowl over a saucepan of simmering water, combine chocolate candy bars and half and half. Stir until completely melted and smooth. Set aside.

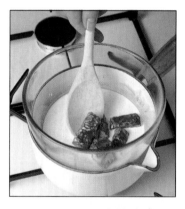

With a knife, cut bananas in half lengthwise. Brush with a little lemon juice to prevent browning. Arrange in 4 long serving dishes and place a layer of strawberries along center of each. Place 2 scoops of ice cream in each dish.

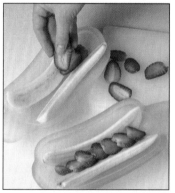

Drizzle fudge sauce over ice cream and bananas, then add a little whipped cream. Finish with a sprinkling of sliced almonds.

Makes 4 servings.

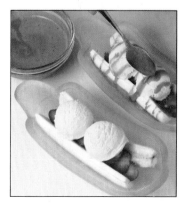

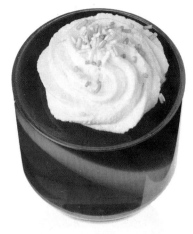

HARLEQUIN JELLIES

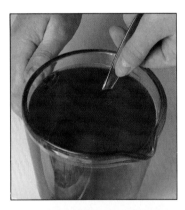

1 (3-oz.) package strawberry- or raspberry-flavored
  gelatin dessert
1 (3-oz.) package lemon- or pineapple-flavored gelatin
  dessert
1 (3-oz.) package black cherry-flavored gelatin dessert
2/3 cup whipping cream
Candy sprinkles, to decorate

Make up the 3 gelatin desserts according to
package directions.

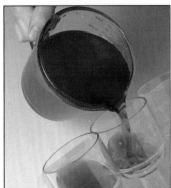

Pour strawberry- or raspberry-flavored gelatin
dessert into 6 tall glasses, each with about 1-
cup capacity: plastic picnic wine glasses are
ideal. Place in refrigerator in a plastic box so
they are tilted; a piece of paper towel roll
placed on the edge will stop glasses from
slipping. Leave until set.

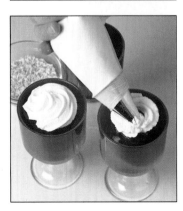

Pour lemon- or pineapple-flavored gelatin
dessert over set red gelatin, then carefully
prop glasses a little more upright, but still on
a tilt. Leave until set. Stand glasses upright
and pour in black cherry-flavored gelatin.
Return to refrigerator to set. Just before
serving, whip cream and pipe on top of each
dessert. Decorate with sprinkles.

Makes 6 servings.

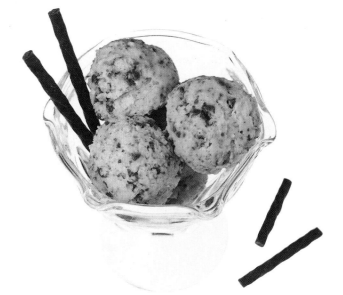

— MINT-CHOC CHIP ICE CREAM —

1 tablespoon custard powder
2 tablespoons sugar
1-1/4 cups milk
1 (6-oz.) can evaporated milk, chilled
Few drops of peppermint extract
Few drops of green food coloring
3 ounces semisweet chocolate, chopped or grated
Chocolate candy sticks, to decorate

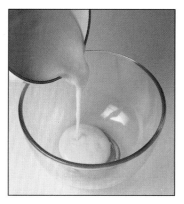

In a small saucepan, blend custard powder and sugar with 2 tablespoons milk. Stir in remaining milk, then cook over low heat until custard thickens, stirring constantly. Remove from heat and pour into a bowl.

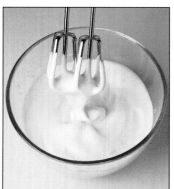

Cover custard's surface with a piece of waxed paper or plastic wrap to prevent a skin from forming. Refrigerate until chilled. In a bowl, beat evaporated milk until very thick. Add peppermint extract and food coloring. Fold into custard, then pour into a shallow freezer-proof container. Place in freezer.

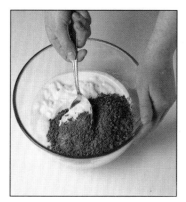

When ice cream is set 1 inch all around edge, turn out into a bowl and beat until smooth. Fold in the chocolate, then return to container and freeze until firm. To serve, transfer ice cream to refrigerator 30 minutes to soften before scooping into bowls or glasses. Decorate with chocolate candies.

Makes 4 to 6 servings.

Note: Instant custard powder is available from specialty food stores.

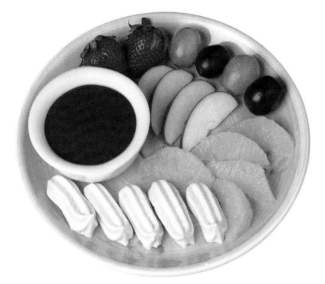

—MILK CHOCOLATE FONDUE—

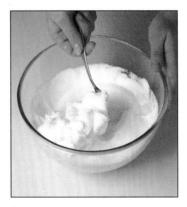

8 ounces milk chocolate
2/3 cup half and half
1/4 cup orange juice
MERINGUES:
2 egg whites
1/2 cup sugar
Selection of fresh fruit, to serve

First, make meringues. Preheat oven to 250F (120C). Line 2 baking sheets with parchment paper. In a bowl, beat egg whites until soft peaks form. Gradually beat in sugar; beat until stiff peaks form.

Spoon meringue mixture into a pastry bag fitted with a small star tip. Pipe small fingers onto lined baking sheets. Bake 1-1/2 to 2 hours, until meringues are dry and crisp. Turn off heat but leave meringues in oven to cool. Peel meringues off parchment paper once they are cool.

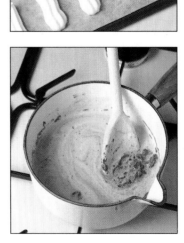

To make fondue, into a small saucepan, break chocolate. Add half and half and orange juice, then place over low heat until chocolate melts, stirring constantly. Pour into a warm serving dish. Serve with meringue fingers and fruit for dipping into chocolate.

Makes 6 to 8 servings.

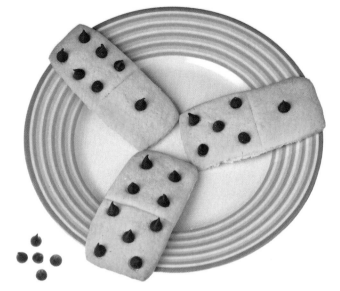

DOMINO COOKIES

2 cups self-rising flour
1/2 cup butter, chilled
1/2 cup sugar
Finely grated zest of 1 lemon
1 small egg, beaten
1 cup semisweet chocolate pieces

Preheat oven to 350F (175C). Into a bowl, sift flour. Cut in butter until mixture resembles bread crumbs. Stir in sugar and lemon zest, then mix in egg to form a dough. Turn out dough onto a floured surface and knead until smooth.

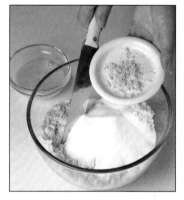

Grease 2 baking sheets. Roll out dough to a rectangle about 1/4-inch thick. With a knife, cut into 3″ x 1-1/2″ bars. With a metal spatula, transfer to baking sheets.

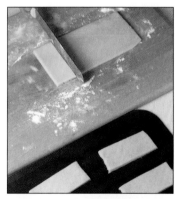

With a knife, mark each cookie crosswise across center. Arrange chocolate pieces on each to resemble domino dots. Bake 12 to 15 minutes, until light brown around edges. Cool slightly on baking sheets, then, with a metal spatula, transfer to a wire rack to cool completely.

Makes about 20.

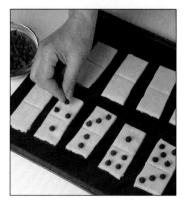

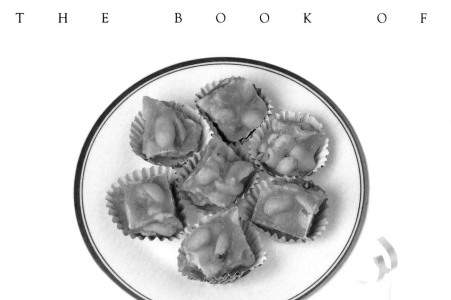

PEANUT BRITTLE

1 heaped cup shelled unsalted peanuts
1-3/4 cups sugar
1/4 cup water
3 tablespoons light corn syrup
2 tablespoons butter
Pinch of baking soda

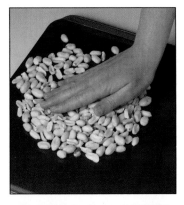

Preheat oven to 275F (135C). Lightly oil an 8-inch square cake pan; set aside. On a baking sheet, toast peanuts about 15 minutes.

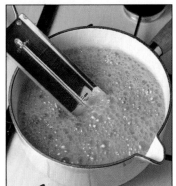

In a heavy-bottomed, medium-size saucepan, combine sugar, water and corn syrup. Cook over medium heat, stirring, until sugar dissolves. Stir in butter, then bring to a boil. Boil rapidly until mixture reaches 300F (150C) on a candy thermometer, or a small amount forms a brittle thread when dropped into a cup of cold water.

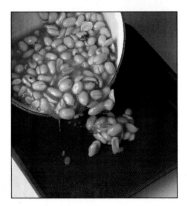

Remove saucepan from heat. Stir in baking soda and toasted peanuts. Pour into oiled pan, stretch slightly with forks, if needed, and cool. When almost set, with an oiled knife, mark into squares. Let set completely. Break into pieces and wrap in colored cellophane, if desired. Store in an airtight container until ready to serve.

Makes about 25 pieces.

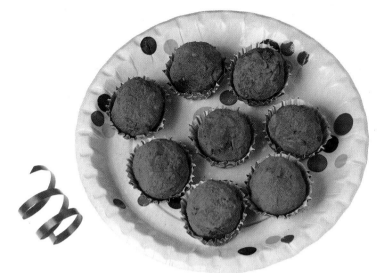

CHOCOLATE BALLS

1/2 cup butter
3 tablespoons light corn syrup
4 ounces semisweet chocolate
3/4 cup chopped dried apricots
1 heaped cup muesli-type cereal
Hot chocolate drink mix

Into a saucepan over low heat, put butter and corn syrup. Heat, stirring, until butter melts.

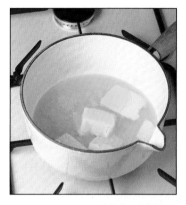

Break in chocolate and melt. Beat together until smooth. Add apricots and cereal; mix together well. Set aside to cool. When cool, refrigerate about 1 hour.

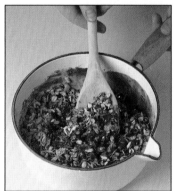

Roll teaspoons of chocolate mixture into balls. Toss in hot chocolate drink mix. Place in petits fours cases. Return to refrigerator until firm.

Makes about 20.

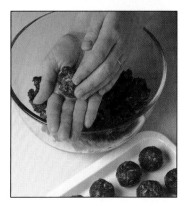

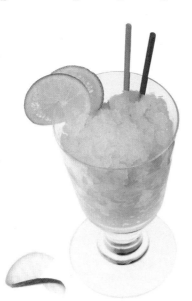

── TROPICAL FRUIT CRUSH ──

1 cup sugar
2 cups water
2 passion fruit
1 ripe mango, peeled and chopped
Juice of 1 orange
Lime slices, to decorate

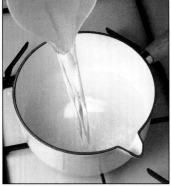

Into a saucepan, put sugar and the 2 cups water. Bring to a boil, then reduce heat and simmer 5 minutes. Set aside to cool.

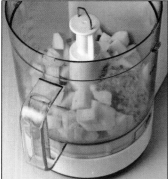

Scoop out flesh from passion fruit. Put into a food processor or blender with mango and orange juice and process until smooth. Pour through a strainer into a bowl; press to remove all juice. Stir in cooled sugar syrup, then pour into a shallow freezerproof tray. Place in freezer.

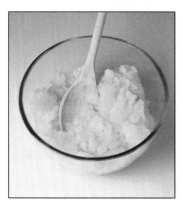

Stir mixture at regular intervals during freezing and continue to freeze until mixture resembles coarse crystals without being frozen solid. Empty into a chilled bowl and crush to break down to small crystals. Return to tray and freeze again until ready to serve. Spoon into glasses and decorate with lime slices.

Makes about 6 servings.

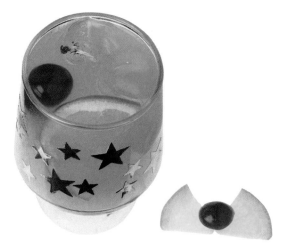

—— SPARKLING FRUIT PUNCH ——

2 oranges
1 (7-oz.) can pineapple pieces in juice
About 10 maraschino cherries
4-1/2 cups orange juice
2 cups pineapple juice
4-1/2 cups lemon-flavored carbonated water
Ice cubes

With a knife, slice oranges, cut in half, and put into a large bowl with pineapple pieces and juice and the cherries.

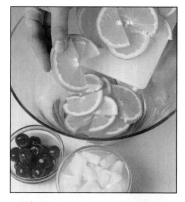

Add orange and pineapple juices and refrigerate until ready to serve.

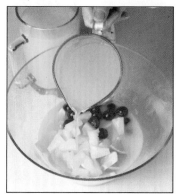

Just before serving, add carbonated water and ice cubes. Serve in glasses, making sure a little fruit is added to each.

Makes about 10 servings.

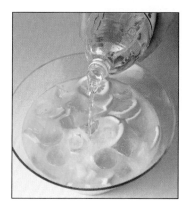

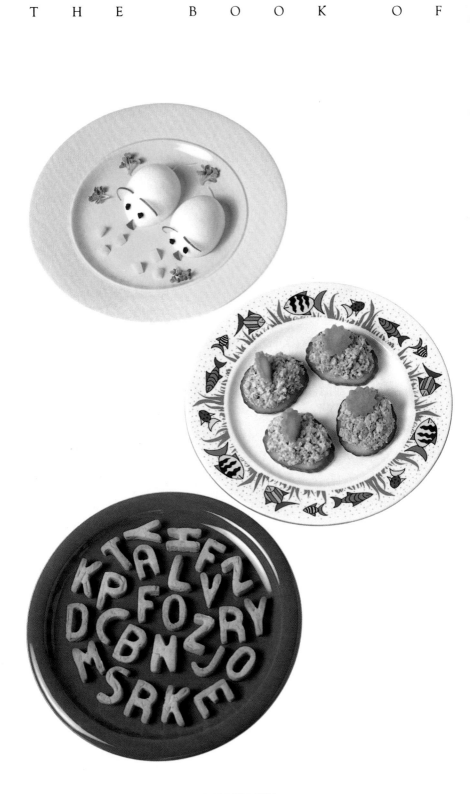

CHEESY MICE
page 29

CUCUMBER SNACKS
page 54

ALPHABET COOKIES
page 27

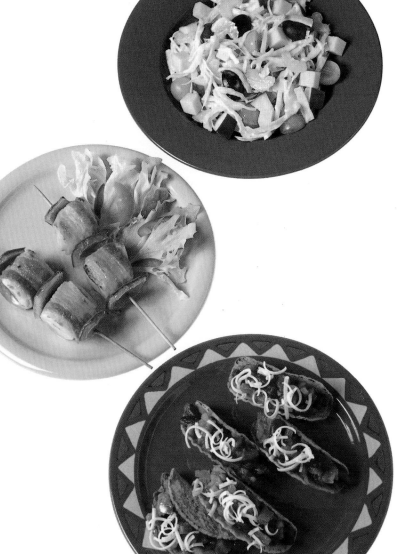

FRUITY CHEESE COLESLAW
page 43

BANANA & BACON KABOBS
page 41

MINI TACOS
page 39

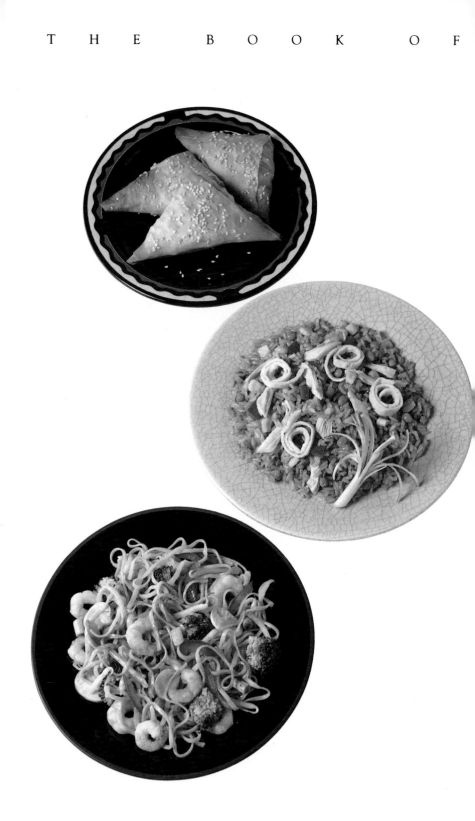

VEGETABLE SAMOSAS
page 74

CHICKEN FRIED RICE
page 81

CHOP SUEY SALAD
page 63

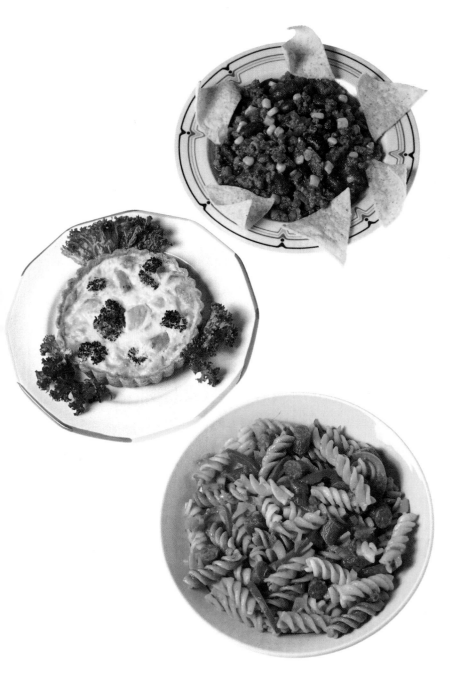

MEXICAN SUPPER
page 75

TURKEY & BROCCOLI QUICHES
page 72

SALAMI PASTA
page 66

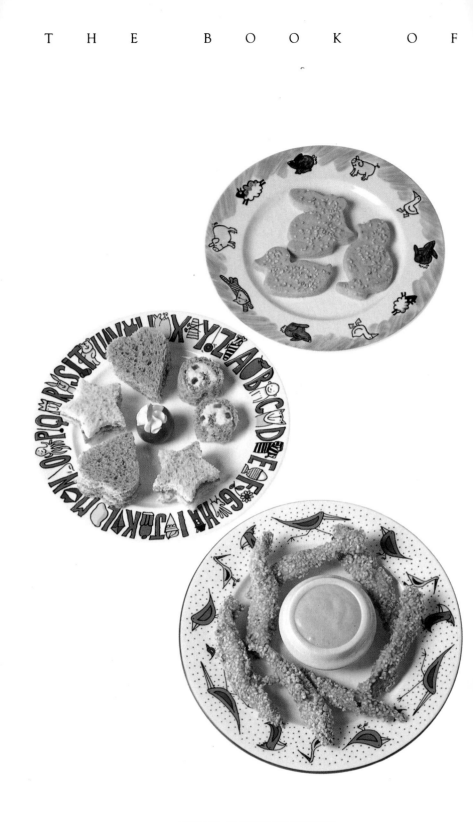

ANIMAL CHEESE CRACKERS
page 91

PARTY SANDWICHES
page 87

SESAME CHICKEN FINGERS
page 92

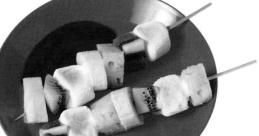

MARSHMALLOW-FRUIT KABOBS
page 100

MERRY MICE CAKES
page 99

TRAFFIC LIGHT COOKIES
page 98

INDEX